DMU 0598871 01 9
WITHDRAWN
DE MONTFORT UNIVERSITY
LIBRARY

AF598694

John Clarkson, Patrick Langdon
and Peter Robinson (Eds)

Designing Accessible Technology

With 85 Figures

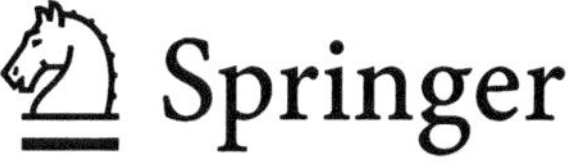

John Clarkson, MA, PhD, CEng, FIEE
Department of Engineering
University of Cambridge
Trumpington Street
Cambridge
CB2 1PZ
UK

Patrick Langdon, BSc, PhD
Department of Engineering
University of Cambridge
Trumpington Street
Cambridge
CB2 1PZ
UK

Peter Robinson, MA, PhD, CEng, FBCS
Computer Laboratory
University of Cambridge
William Gates Building
15 JJ Thomson Avenue
Cambridge
CB3 0FD
UK

British Library Cataloguing in Publication Data
A catalogue record for this book is available from the British Library

Library of Congress Control Number: 2006922619

ISBN-10: 1-84628-364-7 e-ISBN 1-84628-365-5 Printed on acid-free paper
ISBN-13: 978-1-84628-364-2

Printed in Germany

9 8 7 6 5 4 3 2 1

Springer Science+Business Media
springer.com

Designing Accessible Technology

Preface

CWUAAT'06 (incorporating the 6th Cambridge Workshop on Rehabilitation Robotics) is the third of a series of workshops that are held every two years and follows on from the highly successful CWUAAT'02 and CWUAAT'04.

Reflecting the spirit of recent moves to extend the rights for universal accessibility, the new series of workshops is aimed at a broader range of interests, although still with a general focus on product and solution development. Rapid and unprecedented population ageing poses a serious social and economic challenge across the developed world. Shifts in dependency ratios point to escalating welfare and pensions costs which require radical and imaginative responses from Government and industry. The key to this is maintaining a healthy population that is able and willing to work longer before retirement and can remain independent for as long as possible afterwards. A further requirement is to bring disabled people into mainstream life and employment. The CWUAAT workshop has a general focus on product and solution development. Hence the principal requirements for the successful design of assistive and accessible technology are addressed and these range from the identification and capture of the needs of the users, through to the development and evaluation of truly usable and accessible systems for users with special needs.

This book consists of papers received for CWUAAT'06; the contributors representing leading researchers in the fields of Inclusive Design, Rehabilitation Robotics, Universal Access and Assistive Technology. As is usual for CWUAAT, the nature of the contributions has been wide ranging within individual themes and also across the workshop's scope. We believe it is exactly this juxtaposition of research from fields that would not otherwise appear on the same platform, which gives CWUAAT its unique character. It may also be significant that the format of CWUAAT, as a one stream, long presentation workshop held in a single-theatre environment, encourages considered discussion and allows the appraisal of research from a broad range of perspectives, which this year include: multi-institution funded programs into provision for older people; assistive and rehabilitation technology; computer science approaches to inclusive design and rehabilitation; housing design; engineering design of robotic assistance; product design, and social anthropology. All these are united in the common endeavour of improving the design of accessible technology.

The philosophy underlying inclusive design specifically extends the definition of users to include people who are excluded by rapidly changing technology, especially the elderly and ageing, and prioritises the role and value of extreme users in innovation and new product/service development. It also prioritises the context of use, both physical and psychological, and the complexity of interactions between products, services and interfaces in such contexts. Universal access and assistive technology are focussing domains for these priorities. Hence, there is a need to encourage wide-ranging discussion, co-operation and collaboration within and between the universal access and assistive technology research communities in the context of inclusive design and this is met by CWUAAT.

Part I – Design Issues for a More Inclusive World – addresses the maturing field of inclusive design at a theoretical level and in the context of teaching and industry in the UK and abroad.

Part II – Enabling Computer Access And the Development of New Technologies – looks at new technologies that improve accessibility to ITC for older users, the motion impaired and people with Autism, as well as at support tools for designers.

Part III Assistive Technology and Rehabilitation Robotics – showcases research into technology for users with more severe impairments, both for rehabilitation of speech and movement and for improved mobility and dexterity in order to access ICT technology.

Part IV – Understanding Users and Involving Them In the Design Process – reflects on the provision of good quality quantitative and qualitative information about users to designers and on the need to present genuine user needs in the design process.

We would like to thank all those who contributed to the CWUAAT'06 Workshop and to the compilation of this book. Many thanks are also due to all the contributors and the members of the Programme Committee, for the high quality of the reviewing and the resulting papers. Thanks are again due to Christa Croghan and Mari Huhtala, as well as the staff at Fitzwilliam College, who helped to organise and host the workshop.

Pat Langdon, John Clarkson and Peter Robinson
The CWUAAT Editorial Committee
University of Cambridge
April 2006

Cover photograph 'Foam models for Handle with Care' courtesy of Sieberthead and Julia Cassim.

Contents

Part II Enabling Computer Access and the Development of New Technologies

Part III Assistive Technology and Rehabilitation Robotics

Part IV Understanding Users and Involving Them in the Design Process

List of Contributors

Aggarwal N., Alzheimer's Society, Islington, London, UK
Bagnall P., Computing Department, Lancaster University, Lancaster, UK
Bates R., Department of Computing Science, De Monfort University, Leicester, UK
Bichard J-A., The Bartlett, Faculty of the Built Environment, University College, London, UK
Black N., School of Computing and Mathematics, Faculty of Engineering, University of Ulster, Jordanstown, Northern Ireland
Bowen S.J., Art and Design Centre, Sheffield Hallam University, Sheffield, UK
Boyle H., Ergonomics and Safety Research Institute, Loughborough University, Loughborough, Leicestershire, UK
Brooks A., Department of Software and Media Technology, Aalborg University, Esbjerg, Denmark
Chamberlain P.M., Art and Design Centre, Sheffield Hallam University, Sheffield UK
Clarkson P.J., Engineering Design Centre, Department of Engineering, University of Cambridge, Cambridge, UK
Cockerman G., Department of Engineering, Sheffield Hallam University, Sheffield, UK
Conway B., Department of Bioengineering, University of Strathclyde, Glasgow, Scotland, UK
Dautehahn K., Adaptive Systems Research Group, Department of Computer Science, The University of Hertfordshire, Hatfield, Hertfordshire, UK
Davies R., Faculty of Informatics, University of Ulster, Jordanstown, Northern Ireland
Davis.M., Adaptive Systems Research Group, Department of Computer Science, The University of Hertfordshire, Hatfield, Hertfordshire, UK
Dewsbury G., Department of Computer Science, University of Lancaster, Lancaster, UK
Donegan M., ACE Centre, Saddleworth, Lancashire, UK

Dong H., Engineering Design Centre, Department of Engineering, Cambridge University, Cambridge, UK

Driessen B.J.F., TNO TPD, Delft, The Netherlands

Eccleston C., Pain Management Unit, Department of Psychology, University of Bath, Bath, UK

Goodman J., Engineering Design Centre, Department of Engineering, Cambridge University, Cambridge, UK

Gough K.J., Seymourpowell Foresight, London, UK

Greed C., School of Planning and Architecture, University of the West of England (UWE), Bristol, UK

Hammerton J., Centre for Health and Social Care, Sheffield Hallam University, Sheffield, UK

Hansen J.P., Department of Innovation, IT-University, Copenhagen, Denmark

Hanson J., The Bartlett, Faculty of the Built Environment, University College, London, UK

Harding J., Harding Industrial Design, South Moulton, Devon UK

Harris N., Clinical Measurement Department, Royal National Hospital of Rheumatic diseases, Bath, UK

Hood V., Department of Bioengineering, University of Strathclyde, Glasgow, Scotland, UK

Hu H., Department of Computer Science, University of Essex, Colchester, UK

Hughes D.E., Department of Engineering, Sheffield Hallam University, Sheffield, UK

Istance H.O., Department of Computing Engineering, De Monfort University, Leicester, UK

Joyce M.J., Department of Engineering, Lancaster University, Lancashire, UK

King, R., Division of Applied Biomedical Research, King's College, London, UK

Kitchen S., Division of Applied Biomedical Research, King's College, London, UK

Kurniawan S.H., School of Informatics, University of Manchester – UMIST, Manchester, UK

Langdon P.M., Engineering Design Centre, Department of Engineering, University of Cambridge, Cambridge, UK

Lewis T., Engineering Design Centre, Department of Engineering, Cambridge University, Cambridge, UK

Liefhebber F., Delft Centre for Systems and Control, Delft, The Netherlands

Litherland R., Alzheimers Society, Dix's Field, Exeter, Devon, UK

Loudon D., Department of Product Design Engineering, Glasgow School of Art, Glasgow, Scotland, UK

Macdonald A.S., Department of Product Design Engineering, Glasgow School of Art, Glasgow, Scotland, UK

Maguire M., Ergonomics and Safety Research Institute, Loughborough University, Loughborough, Leicestershire, UK

Mayagoita R.E., Division of Applied Biomedical Research, King's College, London, UK

Mawson S.J., Centre for Health and Social care, Sheffield Hallam University, Sheffield, UK

Mitchell V., Ergonomics and Safety Research Institute, Loughborough University, Loughborough, Leicestershire, UK

Monk A.F., Department of Psychology, University of York, Heslington, York, UK
Mountain G.A., Centre for Health and Social Care, Faculty of Health and Well Being, Sheffield Hallam University, Sheffield, UK
Nehaniv C., Adaptive Systems Research Group, Department of Computer Science, The University of Hertfordshire, Hatfield, Hertfordshire, UK
Nicol A.C., Department of Bioengineering, University of Strathclyde, Glasgow, Scotland, UK
Nicolle C., Ergonomics and Safety Research Institute, Loughborough University, Loughborough, Leicestershire, UK
Onditi V., Computing Department, Lancaster University, Lancashire, UK
Paul J.S., Equal Adventure Developments, Aviemore, Scotland, UK
Percival J., School of Health and Social Policy, The Open University, Milton Keynes, UK
Persad U., Engineering Design Centre, Department of Engineering, University of Cambridge, Cambridge, UK
Petersson E., Department of Software and Media Technology, Aalborg University, Esbjerg, Denmark
Potier E., Alzheimer's Society, Kent Region, Chatham, Kent, UK
Powell S., Adaptive Systems Research Group, Department of Computer Science, The University of Hertfordshire, Hatfield, Hertfordshire, UK
Räihä K-J., Department of Computer Sciences, University of Tampere, Finland
Reed D.J., Department of Psychology, University of York, Heslington, York, UK
Roberts P.E., Department of Engineering, Lancaster University, Lancashire, UK
Rouncefield M., Sociology Department, Lancaster University, Lancashire, UK
Rowe P.J., Department of Bioengineering, University of Strathclyde, Glasgow, Scotland, UK
Samuel D., School of Health Professions and Rehabilitation Sciences, University of Southhampton, Southhampton, UK
Savitch N., Centre for HCI Design, City University, London, UK
Simm W.A., Department of Engineering, Lancaster University, Lancashire, UK
Slavík P., Department of Computer Science and Engineering, Czech Technical University, Prague, Czech Republic
Smith M., Nemisys Enterprises Ltd, Hayes, Bedford, UK
Sommerville I., Computing Department, Lancaster University, Lancashire, UK
Sporka A.J., Department of Computer Science and Engineering, Czech Technical University, Prague, Czech Republic
Thean A.H.C., TNO TPD, Delft, The Netherlands
Turner-Smith A., Division of Applied Biomedical Research, King's College, London, UK
Ware P.M., Centre for Health and Social Care, Faculty of Health and Well Being, Sheffield Hallam University, Sheffield, UK
Zaphiris P., Centre for HCI Design, City University, London, UK
Zheng H., School of Computing and Mathematics, Faculty of Engineering, University of Ulster, Jordanstown, Northern Ireland
Zhou H., Department of Computer Science, University of Essex, Colchester, Essex UK

Part I

Design Issues for a More Inclusive World

Chapter 1

The Inclusive Challenge: A Multidisciplinary Educational Approach

A.S. Macdonald

1.1 Introduction

With the occurrence of a rapidly ageing population, the issue of universal access and inclusivity is a challenging and complex one: this will require a coherent multidisciplinary approach. Technologists and engineers will undoubtedly help find some parts of the solutions to accessibility, but whereas people previously had to adapt to technologies, technologies will now have to come closer to people. To achieve this, a better understanding of what is acceptable in terms of the way that the technology is delivered is required. To achieve this within educational curricula it will be necessary to create space to work with other disciplines.

In this paper, the author argues the case for a more strategic approach to education involving a broad range of disciplines representing future policy makers, technologists and bureaucrats. He argues that the value and relevance of the methods, examples and processes of an inclusive design educational approach should be applied across a wider range of disciplines than solely design. One challenge facing design educationalists is how to introduce and deliver a coherent 'inclusive' design curriculum based on the growing body of recommendations and increasingly available resources.

This paper compares and discusses, through case studies, the relative successes of two different approaches, both developed by the author, and their relevance to the field of inclusive technologies. The author, who has twenty years experience of teaching design almost totally devoted to design and engineering students, also discusses the core content of the curricula for each of the two cases and their impact on the respective groups of students' perceptions of 'inclusive', assistive and accessible solutions.

1.2 Questions Arising

As the demographics of an ageing population will increasingly present us with some tough design challenges, are we being strategic enough in our use of design education in anticipating and preparing for these challenges? If the benefits of an inclusive approach to design are to be as effective as they will need to be, should design educationalists consider widening their teaching audience to include non-design students? Design is 'just' one of a number of key areas of expertise that influence the shape and accessibility of our built environment. Is there a need for a greater understanding of the contribution that an inclusive approach to design can offer when working alongside these other fields?

1.3 Two Approaches

Two cases will be discussed. In the first case an inclusive approach to design has been embedded in an UK design-centred engineering curriculum at undergraduate level. In the second, this approach has been modified for a wide range of non-design graduate students in Japan through a short, intensive stand-alone course. For each case, an outline of the content of the curriculum is discussed, as well as the approach and implications resulting from these two experiences.

1.3.1 Case 1: Inclusive Design in a Design-centred Engineering Curriculum

There is an emerging debate about what should constitute an inclusive design syllabus and some excellent resources and recommendations already exist (IDCnet, 2004). In the first case discussed, that of the Glasgow Product Design Engineering (PDE) course, (run jointly between the Glasgow School of Art and the University of Glasgow) there is no separate 'inclusive design' syllabus as such due to the existing pressures of a demanding and accredited engineering curriculum and design studio project timetable, but instead one where an inclusive agenda is developed within the cohort group. Such an approach requires, *e.g.,* personal individual (staff) commitment to that agenda, politicking to demonstrate its benefits both to staff and students, separate briefings, access to self-learning materials, and appropriate strategies and guidelines for designing.

Fortunately, this agenda has now been enthusiastically adopted and embedded as a structured approach in the ethos of the department, facilitated by a steadily growing interest in medical, welfare, rehabilitation and assistive product areas. This has promoted beneficial collaborations with new (to the department) disciplines such as healthcare, rehabilitation and clinical medicine.

Through a series of briefings, the 'inclusive design' syllabus in this case covers context (change in population demographic, lifestyle and technological trends), 'people' models (how one thinks about a range of different capabilities and how these differ from individual to individual, and dynamically with age or illness), inclusive, or universal, design principles (with which to evaluate concepts, designs and services), and a typology of user research methods (as involvement with users from the earliest stages of the design process is crucial for successful, usable, and desirable design proposals). Additionally, access to self-learning resources, case studies and exemplars, such as found in the excellent web-site developed by the Royal Society of Arts (RSA), is invaluable.

This approach appears to have been fruitful as it has achieved success in the area of inclusive design in student design competitions at a UK national level. PhD level research activity has also emerged, *e.g.,* ranging from 'inclusive' software tools for designers (Rowe *et al.*, 2005) that provide a bridge between biomechanical data and its value in designing products for an ageing population, to design tools for exploring issues relating to the (non-) adoption of technologies by different generations – the 'generation effect' (Lim and Macdonald, 2005).

1.3.2 Case 2: Inclusive Design for Future Policy Makers

In the second case study, the central concern is one of how to engender sufficient understanding of the value and efficacy of an inclusive approach to design for all aspects of the built environment, in future societal policy makers, in shapers of technological strategies, and in the future commissioners of design. This case discusses the Master's level Inclusive Design course run in three successive years (2003-2005) at the Center for Global Education and Research at the Ritsumeikan (Rits) University in Kyoto, Japan. The Rits does not have design as a subject specialisation or department as such.

Here, in an enlightened and strategic approach commissioned by the Rits, inclusive design is seen as one crucial area of expertise, amongst others, required to inform a class of enlightened techno-bureaucrats with the awareness and knowledge to anticipate and prepare for emergent and pressing societal needs, *e.g.,* in the areas of governance, welfare, security, technology and design.

Masters students from a wide range of disciplines which have included law, sociology, health studies, core ethics and frontier sciences, policy science, business administration, marketing, human (interface) engineering, and mechanical engineering elect for this one-week intensive lecture-, assignment- and workshop-based 'inclusive design' course.

Again, for this to succeed, such an approach requires individual commitment to the promotion of the 'inclusive' agenda, to communicate the value of the course both to staff and students, and to attract elective participants.

Here the curriculum is similar in some of its content to that of Case 1, *i.e.,* context (but with greater emphasis on the nature and scale of the emerging challenge in order to highlight the need for a strategic approach through a number of specialist fields working together), 'people' models, universal design principles, user research methods, and with access to the same sorts of on-line self-learning resources as in Case 1. Design process, which is familiar through the normal curriculum in Case 1, is introduced in the Case 2 curriculum to illustrate, through a number of exemplars, how designers can embody principles, services, and technologies in a 'humanised' (Macdonald, 2003) or user-centric way. One major component of the Case 2 curriculum is a forum for discussing issues of *e.g.*, enabling, disabling, acceptability, inclusivity and exclusivity, as the effectiveness of a response to a situation or a problem may depend on whether this is in a 'medical' or 'social' mode (see further discussion below). This is facilitated through 'workshop' style activities, including the use of empathetic methods such as compromising capabilities by taping up joints to modify dexterity and sensitivity, and the use of special spectacles that simulate different types of conditions affecting sight (see Figure 1.1).

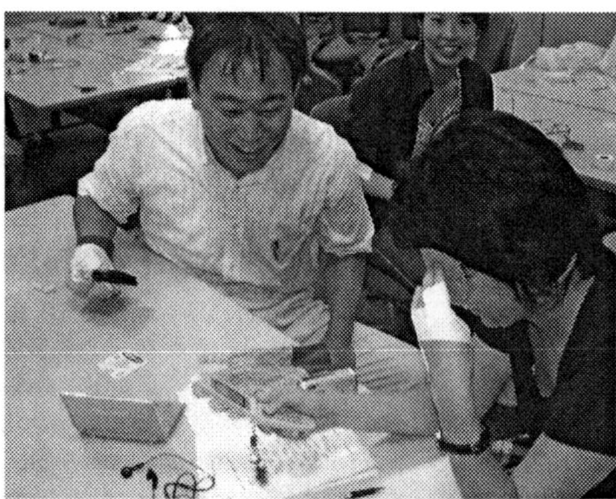

Figure 1.1. Students from mixed disciplines at the Rits, Kyoto, using empathetic methods to understand capability limitations when interfacing with products

1.4 Discussion

The metrics for evaluating the second case are harder to define as any benefits accruing will not be as immediately – or tangibly – obvious as in the first, although feedback has been solicited through questionnaires and self-evaluation forms at the completion of the Rits courses, and reference to this is made later. The following discussion compares outcomes common to both approaches and those that are unique to each. In both cases, limited time is available for exploring inclusive issues, context, values, ideals, methods, models and exemplars, but within each case, a heightened awareness of inclusive design issues and the need for a more inclusive approach to shaping our environment has undoubtedly been observed in participating students.

1.4.1 Case 1: Glasgow

In the case of an established course such as Glasgow's PDE, 'inclusivity', like the issue of 'sustainability', has had to be embedded into an existing and full design engineering curriculum. Activity at senior undergraduate level tends to be more individually based in the form of a major project over a single session. The single discipline of expertise, *i.e.,* PDE in this case, requires that a 'product' outcome is delivered - so there is an element of expediency in the approach, and the responses tend to be (but are not exclusively) more in the 'medical' mode. The medical model of disability and ageing implies that people are disabled as a consequence of their own condition, and seeks to either remedy or correct the impairment through medication, rehabilitation and surgery *etc.,* or offers adaptive aids and equipment as a physical remedy (Clarkson *et al.,* 2003). The student's habitual approach and response is modified only to a limited extent by contact with other disciplines and this contact is again 'expedient' in nature – being driven by the need for an informed and inclusive 'product' outcome.

In this first case, students consolidate their field of professional expertise and are able to embody inclusive principles and ideals in realisable, manufacturable product solutions that have the ability to make a measurable difference to the quality of a person's life. Examples might include innovative surgical, rehabilitation, self-medication, or assistive devices. Figure 1.2 illustrates a good 'product' response to the problem of ill or elderly people unable to attend a dentist's practice, in the form of a portable dental surgery. Here, the case is made that technology can, *e.g.,* utilise inclusive design thinking to help extend social provision.

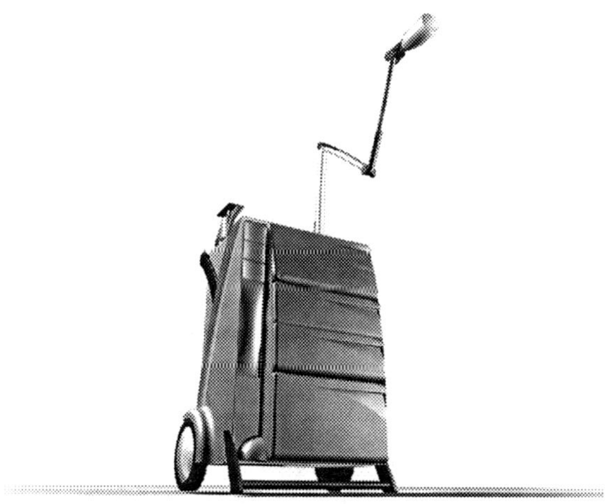

Figure 1.2. Portable dental surgery, Scott Maguire, PDE 2003, Glasgow

1.4.2 Case 2: Kyoto

In the second case, at the Rits, the Inclusive Design course opens up, within the limitations of 15 sessions over five days, a new 'space' in the student's typical educational curriculum to address a shared – and in this case, a pressing - societal issue, that of an ageing population. This space provides the opportunity for potentially any discipline to benefit from the knowledge, perceptions and responses of others, and allows a certain freedom for participants to respond to the issues being addressed in previously untried ways, perhaps not habitually associated with their own discipline. Here, there is no requirement for a specific 'designed' outcome as such, rather to develop a critical view of the existing built environment and its infrastructure, and associated products, interfaces and services, and to highlight opportunities for improvement that could be service-based, or policy-based, or product-based, or indeed a mixture of these.

The 'vehicle' to develop this critical and reflective approach is an assignment themed on 'the modern journey' (MIRAKEL, 2002) (Figure 1.3), a detailed photographic critique of the process of making a journey by various modes of public transport across a city, commenting on products, interfaces, environments and services. It is used as a means to identify the complexity of inter-related issues, and for the combination of disciplines required to address these in creating accessible civic environments. This provides the means for both a tangible analysis and addressing of the issues raised in the accompanying lecture series (which provides core information on relevant issues, and exemplars) and group discussions on the one hand, and the development of a personal 'portfolio' or 'agenda' on the other. Here, the responses tend to be more – but not exclusively - in the 'social' mode which sees people as disabled or enabled by the social context in which they function and proposes that changes in the social context or environment can remove or alleviate disability (Clarkson *et al.,* 2003).

In this case, one has to take care that students do not think they have to provide 'designs' as such because the course leader in this case is a design lecturer and is thought to expect these, but even if this is the case, they will have had some, albeit limited, experience of another professional domain, in this case, design.

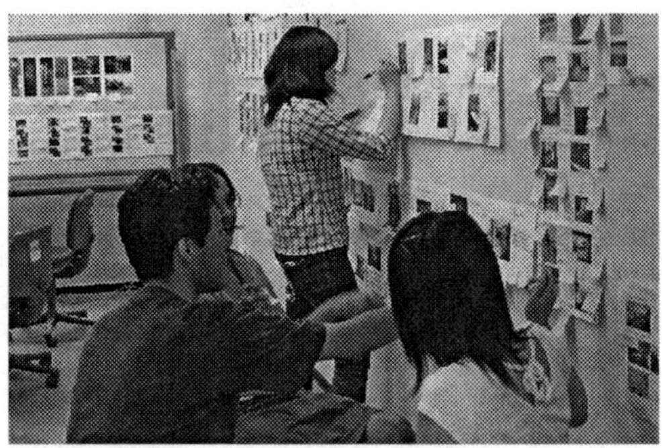

Figure 1.3. Students from mixed disciplines at the Rits, Kyoto, critiquing 'the modern journey' photographic assignment

In the Rits case, students are able to significantly develop their awareness of the relationship between their professional field of expertise and the others participating, and to understand that in tackling the complexity of the 'inclusive' challenges facing society there is a common agenda shared amongst different professional fields, and that to achieve progress, this requires a coordinated approach with a shared vision. Here, each student is able to offer a response to the inclusive challenge informed by their own discipline but in a context that recognises that there are many other modes of responding to the same issue, whether that be, *e.g.,* a product, a service, a policy, or a combination of all of these. In this case, the 'total package' of what is required for an inclusive or accessible solution is less constrained by the strictures of a particular discipline, but one can develop an appreciation of how best to introduce *e.g.,* an assistive technology within a civic service.

Feedback solicited through questionnaires from the Rits students at the end of the courses gives some indication of the perceived value of the course to these students. Clearly evident in the 2005 course, where more 'workshop' sessions were utilised, was the fact that non-design students are perfectly capable of presenting coherent service-based or product-based concepts when introduced to design tools such as 'brainstorming', 'scenario-building' and 'concept visualisation': Figure 1.4 shows an MBA student's concept for an electronic inclusive business trip pass. It appears that students at the Rits do not normally have the opportunity for inter-disciplinary collaboration – "it differs greatly from the usual class form of the university" and that group work is not common "learning ... with classmates [belonging to] various research courses [gives an] enhanced class." In response to an empathetic methods session (students were asked to tape up their fingers to reduce mobility and sensitivity when using a mobile phone (Figure 1.2), one policy science masters student reported that *"the inconvenience was able to be actually experienced ... and it became an experience beyond price".*

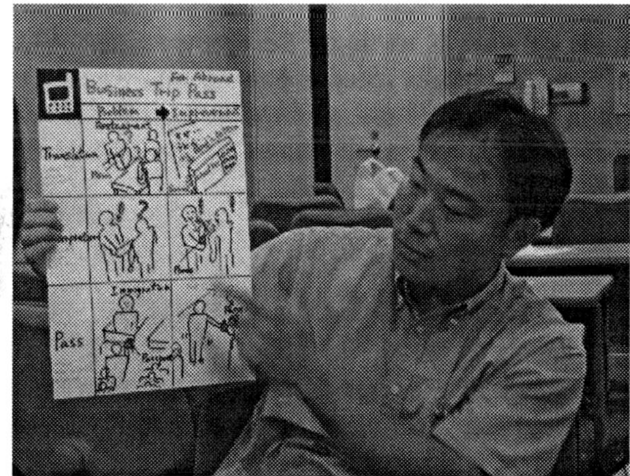

Figure 1.4. Concept for an electronic inclusive business trip pass, Shinichi Fujita, MBA student, Rits 2005

1.5 The Strategic Challenge

Society will always require individuals with the professional design and engineering skills to translate people's needs into the tangible, realisable products and services required for the 'made' world for our daily lives. These will need to be humanely designed, embody accessible and inclusive features, and be pleasurable and life-enhancing to use.

At the same time, we are faced with an enormous demographic shift that presents us, in the developed world, with a population that will have a greater range of capabilities and requirements than ever before. Two thirds of the world's population will live in cities by 2030 (Reader, 2004), and this will require us to think about how the environment and services in these cities should be shaped so that we create inclusive, 'intentional' cities rather than exclusive 'accidental' ones.

This author argues that there is a strong case for exposing those who will never consider being designers *per se,* to the models, processes and methods of design to provide insights that will enable them to use design and designers more effectively as part of a wider societal strategy. However, the inclusive issues facing society suggest we should consider how we should do this with some urgency.

The Rits experience highlights the fact that, certainly in a country such as Japan where inclusive (or as it is preferred to be known 'universal') design is a much more widely appreciated concept in the community as a whole, there is an interest in and appetite for at least a greater appreciation and application of the inclusive design agenda amongst a range of different professional sectors such as those already mentioned. The extent to which the population in Japan at large is familiar with concepts such as 'barrier-free' or 'universal' design is impressive due to the promotion of this agenda at a civic, as well as a national level. Japanese industry has also heavily promoted the universal agenda, so its strategic role and value is much better understood and utilised than in the UK (Macdonald, 2006). While there are some excellent Inclusive Design educational resources and guidelines available arising out of work done in the European context, (IDCnet, 2004), in the Rits case it has been important to take into account the cultural differences in Japanese society, in the educational environment, and within the Rits university itself, and to clearly understand its objectives in fostering and promoting this type of activity.

1.6 Observations and Conclusions

The Rits case illustrates that elements of a design-led educational approach have a value to students of subject disciplines other than solely those being trained for some form of design profession or activity.

The experience of introducing masters level students who have had no previous formal design education or exposure to structured thinking on inclusive design and issues of inclusivity has demonstrated that even through limited exposure, such as the short intensive course at the Rits, a more considered, person-centred approach can be fostered in a range of disciplines. *"At first, I thought that old people were the target of the research, but now I think the problem is also ... with young people"* (mechanical engineering master), *"I consulted my aged grandmother, and was able to understand that our not being able to do [tasks] naturally becomes difficult when eyesight and hearing failed...[something we do not] usually notice"* (policy science master).

If more design educators were working across a wider spectrum of disciplines than solely the professional development of young designers, this would help to ensure that those emerging design professionals with their new skills sets find improved opportunities to attain the inclusive ideal through more enlightened policy makers and commissioners of design. It also suggests that within existing subject discipline courses, a less 'expediency-driven' space in the curriculum needs to be opened up for a freer and more critical examination of issues involving a wider range of disciplines, allowing a wider range of appropriate modes of response to address these strategically.

There are a great many developments in new technologies that have the potential to improve the quality of life, especially for an ageing population. During a three-month Fellowship in 2004 to research Inclusive Design and Technologies in Japan, the author visited a number of technology and engineering research laboratories in Nagoya, Osaka and Kyoto, and Tokyo. The preoccupations of their professional field naturally precluded them from a more human-centred approach to technological application, but the majority of the engineers and technologists interviewed had a strong interest in the potential of design to 'humanise' the applications of their research and to provide an appropriate human interface at point of contact. They also tended to be aware of the inclusive agenda. What is also interesting is that in many of the technological companies in Japan, the universal approach has created new processes, new tools, and a new approach, reflecting a greater empathy with end users, that is much closer to their customers' values and to satisfying their lifestyle goals than previously (Macdonald, 2006).

Although Case 2 experience demonstrates that the approach has an application to a wide range of subject disciplines, in the context of assistive technological approaches specifically, the author concludes that more of those working in assistive technology and related fields would benefit from exposure to even a short course such as described in Case 2 at the Rits. One might just witness, as a result, more technological products emerge on to the market which are more user friendly, more accessible, and more inclusive. This would help develop a mode of thinking about how to better apply technological innovation to this pressing societal issue of an ageing population, and to help transform something that is regarded here as a potential societal burden, to something – as it is now beginning to be regarded in Japan - as a real opportunity. This would help extend the recommendations in the UK Design Council's 'Living Longer' agenda for plugging the knowledge gaps in inclusive design (Coleman, 2000).

1.7 Acknowledgements

My sincere thanks to the dedicated staff and students in Product Design Engineering at Glasgow School of Art and at the Ritsumeikan University, Kyoto. Also to the Japan Foundation, the Royal Academy of Engineering UK, and the Center for Global Education and Research at the Ritsumeikan University, Kyoto, Japan, for supporting aspects of this research.

1.8 References

Clarkson PJ, Coleman R, Keates S, Lebbon C (eds.) (2003) Inclusive design: design for the whole population. Springer, London, UK

Coleman R (2000) Living longer: the new context for design. Design Council, London

Lim CS, Macdonald AS (2005) Eras, generations and new technologies. Gerontechnology 3(4): 213

Macdonald AS (2003) Humanising technology. In: Clarkson PJ *et al.* (eds.) Inclusive design: design for the whole population. Springer, London, UK

Macdonald AS (2006) Universal design in Japanese technological industries. In: Clarkson PJ *et al.* (eds.) Designing accessible technology. Springer, London, UK

IDCnet (2004) Identifying core knowledge and skills sets for model curricula: IST-2001-38786. Update 2004, European Design for All e-Accessibility Network. Available at: http://www.edean.org/docareasigs/Curricula_on_DfA/IDCnet%20Deliverables/IDCnet_D3.2.1.pdf

MIRAKEL (2002) The modern journey – from another perspective. MIRAKEL Film and TV AB, The Nordic Council, Sweden

Reader J (2004) Cities. William Heinemann, London, UK

Rowe PJ, Hood V, Loudon D, Samuel D, Nicol AC *et al.* (2005) Calculating and presenting biomechanical functional demand in older adults during activities of daily living. In: Proceedings of IASTED BioMech2005, Benidorm, Spain

RSA (2005) Available at: http://www.inclusivedesign.org.uk

Chapter 2

Universal Design in Japanese Technological Industries

A.S. Macdonald

2.1 Introduction

This author argues that an inclusive approach to design offers a better way of designing *per se* and also offers a new design vocabulary to help technological industries understand and better relate to the values and goals of their end-users. Over the past decade or so, research into the area of inclusive (or universal) design and design for ageing has provided the catalyst for the emergence of a rich resource of new models and approaches which together begin to suggest a new paradigm for designing. This is evident not only in academia, but also in industry. Nowhere is this more evident than in the recent approaches taken by Japanese industries involved in the production of technological consumer products. Whereas legislative push provides certain 'barrier-free' modifications and advances in the public realm, and promotes personal rights to accessible products and services, it is the market pull experienced by these industries that is responsible for increasing numbers of inclusive products appearing on the marketplace, enhancing quality-of-life and supporting lifestyle goals. This discussion draws from literature and papers published by and interviews with individuals in a number of Japanese companies. The terms 'inclusive' and 'universal' are here used synonymously.

2.2 Inclusive Tools and Resources

Research on ageing and inclusive design over the past decade has provided a number of new models and approaches for design and industry. Amongst these are those that provide a more inclusive approach to anthropometric modelling; models describing needs and capabilities; principles and guidelines; and improved processes, such as co-creation and management approaches.

Taken as a whole, this body of recent research material constitutes a vastly improved 'toolkit' for the processes and means of designing. Taken together, the outcomes begin to suggest a new paradigm for how we think about designing and the end users, one of socially responsible design imbued with implicit and explicit humanitarian values.

More than this, they also provide those businesses and industries creating technological products with a much more comprehensive understanding of the users and their values, with a richer vocabulary for understanding, discussing and promoting the humane applications of technologies within a consumerist society.

> *"...people used to have to come close to technology, but now technology is coming closer to people."*
>
> (Hosoyama, 2004)

In Japan, the business community has realised that this approach is not only a better way to design, but is also an approach whose values seem to resonate with those of an evolving and increasingly diverse and sophisticated marketplace.

2.3 Legislative Push and Market Pull

Without detailing the historical process, general awareness in the population at large of 'universal access' or 'barrier-free' provision in Japan has been heightened through various forms of legislation including 'barrier-free' requirements in the public realm. In Japan, a strong lobby for the visually impaired has resulted in 'tactile pathways' on pavements, 'tactile points' on electrical goods, Braille signage in elevators and handrails, sonic signals at road crossings and station entrances, and auditory information on public transportation for the blind. However, total blindness represents but a small proportion of those with vision deficiencies who need to be served by products and services (Kawahara, 2005a). There is a large - and growing - range of diverse capabilities that require to be catered for in the population at large due the ageing demographic and it is difficult to see how this can be met by legislative means alone. In Japan this has been understood as a consumer issue:

> *"It's a consumer market driven issue. Its focus is not specifically on people with disabilities, but all people. It actually assumes the idea that everybody has a disability."*
>
> (JIPRI, 2000)

However, it is the recent response from Japanese industry to this 'universal challenge' that is of interest and is now discussed in more detail. This response needs to be seen against the backdrop of a rapidly (now 'super-') ageing society and a declining birth rate, and in the spending power of this now significant sector of the population.

2.4 Universal Values Made Explicit

The adoption of 'inclusive' or 'universal' principles has been, to an extent, accelerated by the recently (2003) established International Association of Universal Design (IAUD) which in 2005 had some 135 companies in its membership. IAUD Chairman (of the Council) Kazuo Toda stated that:

> *"the Japanese House of Councillors passed a 'resolution on the promotion of a Universally Accessible Society' in June 2004. This resolution takes a step further from the standpoints of welfare for the disabled and barrier-free promotion that were in existence in the past, and indicates a stance by the state in favour of creating an integrated social environment that operates from the viewpoint of universal design."*
>
> (IAUD, 2005)

2.4.1 Developing Principles

This acknowledgement of the societal context, and the concern for humane applications of technologies is one that has become explicit in the literature and emerging practice of Japanese companies involved in the production of technological goods. For example, Matsushita/Panasonic states that the:

> *"universal design concept seeks to develop products which will help create inclusive societies in which all people can enjoy high-amenity lifestyles."*
>
> (Matsushita, 2004)

Depending on which of its sources one consults, Matsushita/Panasonic uses five, six, or eight principles or customer-centred points to be considered when taking a 'universal' approach to design. Their 2004 report goes on to say:

> *"...while technical innovation is constantly advancing, it is also creating a divide. Matsushita believes that bringing prosperity, fun, and comfort to more people through products and services is a corporate social responsibility."... "providing consideration to more people through products and services in an attempt to establish enriched lifestyles in which more people live in comfort."*
>
> (Matsushita, 2004)

The broad spectrum of individuals that make up society is also acknowledged in Toshiba's philosophy which recognises:

> *"...the old and the young, the fit and the frail, different people, all with different needs and lifestyles. Our products are designed to be shared by everybody, easy for us all to use."*
>
> (Toshiba, 2004)

2.4.2 From Guidelines and Principles to Standards

Fujitsu recognised that:

> *"as the degree of IT utilization increases in our daily lives, universal design is becoming an essential approach if we are to create a convenient and value-added lifestyle for as many people as possible. We also strive to realise universal design 'from the customer's point of view' to contribute to the success of the customer's business." Fujitsu "introduced the Universal Design Product Guidelines in 2002, which lists eight consumer-centred points to be considered at the product development stage."*
>
> (Fujitsu, 2004)

From this standpoint, Fujitsu began basic training in the company in 2003. It has introduced two types of Universal Design (UD) 'recognitions'. One is 'UD Approved Products', products with industry-leading levels of UD adoption, and these are marked by a UD symbol. The other type is the 'UD Conscious Product' – products meeting in-house standards. It should be said that Fujitsu is not only thinking about the 'market out there', but how it can increase accessibility and usability, and user-friendliness, *i.e.* 'inclusivity', for its own company employees.

Because Japanese industries appear to share their findings and appear to publish much more openly than their counterparts in the UK and Europe, many of the companies in the IAUD membership have advanced policies of awareness-raising, design tools and methods, and universal standards within their companies. For example, the Japanese Industrial Standards (JIS) officially announced a standard (JIS X 8341) for promoting the UD of products and services in the information field, and have gone on to suggest to the ISO that UD be standardised, and that the IAUD should assist in that process (Kato and Iwazaki, 2005).

This has also permeated to universities at a teaching level, where companies will take their experience in universal design back into higher education. For instance, the author attended a critique at Kobe Design University involving a small group of final year undergraduate product design students who were addressed by a mixed group of industrial designers with universal design remits from Saxa, Mitsubishi, Oki, Canon, NEC, and Panasonic. These were all members of the Communications and Information network Association of Japan (CIAJ) which together had developed a shared universal design approach.

2.4.3 Transforming Principles and Standards into Products: Toyota

One can observe the maturing fruits of this approach in recent products. The case study of, *e.g.*, the development of the Toyota *Raum* (Macdonald, 2005) launched in 2003, interestingly reveals Toyota's explicit adoption of embedded universal principles in one of their vehicles for the first time, and in their *Porte*, launched in 2004, one can begin to see an increasingly sophisticated understanding of how these principles might sit in a wider societal context. Toyota may not be the only manufacturer to be pursuing this line of development, but these two vehicles serve as particularly valuable exemplars.

These designs have been achieved through an iterative user-centred process, and by developing concepts by means of multiple user scenarios throughout the design process. These methods were not in place in Toyota before 1997 (Ohshima, 2004). Not only do the designs of both these Toyota vehicles meet the stringent engineering challenges of passenger safety and performance, and meet the testing ergonomic requirements of functionality, usability and user-friendliness, but, for the *Raum,* Toyota developed two indices, an 'ergo-index', and a 'situation suitability index', together with a 'spiral-up' development process to enhance the universal design qualities of its vehicles.

> *"In alignment with the principles of universal design, we have adopted a short Japanese slogan* an-raku-tan *to help maintain focus of many designers on the overall design...* an-raku-tan *means peace of mind, pleasure and singularity, but also suggests the ideas of soothing, safe, affordable, easy, fun, beautiful, elemental and simple."*
>
> (Atsumi, Kanamori and Misugi, 2005)

What is interesting here is the emergence, in what was previously a predominantly engineering-technical-production-dominated sphere, of a new user-centred vocabulary based on human values and goals.

The engineering involved that facilitated the major innovations (*e.g.* the removal of the door-pillar on the passenger side to create a 1.5 metre-wide opening in the *Raum*) is accomplished and innovative, and one which has been much emulated since, but it was the human and social need that drove the innovation. This design is not about stylistic options, but true accessibility and flexibility of space, to allow both individual customisation and flexibility amongst a number of users whose needs are diverse. However, it is worth noting that the marketing of the 'universal' qualities of the *Raum* was fairly explicit, and consequently the product may have tended to be linked, at least in consumers' minds, with disability and ageing, and with the 'barrier-free' legislation then recently introduced into the public domain:

> *"... the Raum had put emphasis on the older and disabled user and as a consequence this had not sold well."*
>
> (Hosoyama, 2004)

By contrast, Toyota's *Porte*, launched in August 2004, as a second-generation 'universal' vehicle, was promoted much more as a lifestyle car:

> *"...a smart life supporter"... "a new category family vehicle like causal wear."*
>
> (Ohshima, 2004)

The website format for the Porte is based around lifestyle: this can be run as a simple animation showing multi-mode use of the vehicle. In the various scenarios that can be played out on this website, disability access, whether by wheelchair or other requirement, is seen as 'just' another option that the design of the vehicle can accommodate, alongside surfboards, gardening supplies, groceries, and, culturally important in Japan, one can emerge from the vehicle with an already opened umbrella to protect oneself from sun or rain. As a design, the *Porte* is shorter but higher than the *Raum*, with a narrower power-assisted side door, one that can be remote-controlled, and with a flat floor.

Interestingly, in the *Porte*, the awareness of requirements for ageing and disability have been assimilated into the overall design process of a vehicle which has also a degree of enjoyment and fun associated with it – an important lifestyle ingredient whether one is aged, disabled, or not. What we may be seeing in this exemplar is the first fruits of a new and much improved way of designing that has assimilated universal principles through a sophisticated array of user-focussed design tools and models, and a more mature understanding of the market.

2.5 Conclusions

One is beginning to see quite noticeably in Japan, through a mixture of legislative push and market pull, the creation of a heightened awareness of inclusive values amongst the population at large, whether private citizen, student, academic, industrialist or indeed civic administration. This was concluded from numerous conversations and interviews conducted over a three-month period from September to December 2004. In the summer of 2005, Kyoto city published a widely available civic 'manifesto' embracing seven universal design principles which it will use to shape its public realm.

Industries creating technological consumer products have had a significant role to play in this process, and have meaningfully embraced the inclusive agenda and its challenges. The significant demographic shift and projections of the ageing profile in Japan have stimulated, if not forced, strategic inclusive approaches supported by an array of inclusive models, tools, and processes that acknowledge the needs, values, and lifestyle goals of the end users.

A new generation of young design managers in these technological companies can be seen developing tools of their own, and proactively sourcing, internationally, the fruits of academic research in this area, evaluating these and integrating these, if and as appropriate, into company practices. Although the companies are individually competitive, they have realised there is mutual advantage in sharing approaches and aspirations through fora such as the IAUD, or the CIAJ, understanding that by mutual cooperation, the game-plan for Japanese products and the number of these on the market that serve the inclusive needs of their society will be at a much higher level than their foreign competitors (Kawahara, 2005b).

With their 'super-ageing' society, Japanese industry has had to act to address the challenges brought by their rapidly changing population, economic and social demographic, and in so doing has provided a timely and valuable exemplar for those regions that will imminently, and unavoidably, have to face a similar challenge.

2.6 Acknowledgements

The author gratefully acknowledges the assistance of the Japan Foundation, the Ritsumeikan University's (Kyoto) Discovery Research Laboratory, and the Royal Academy of Engineering for supporting this research, and the many individuals in companies and universities who gave freely of their time in many stimulating discussions.

2.7 References

Atsumi B, Kanamori H, Misugi K (2005) Toyota's program for universal design in vehicle development. Gerontechnology 3(4): 228

Kato K, Iwazaki A (2005) Fujitsu's activities for universal design. Fujitsu Science and Technology Journal 41(1): 3–9

Kawahara K (2005a) Considerations in universal design in terms of physical function characteristics of the aged. Gerontechnology 3(4): 211

Kawahara K (2005b) The author in conversation with Keiji Kawahara, Director, KID Studio Corporation, Nagoya, Japan

Fujitsu (2004) Fujitsu company report 2004. Available at: http://www.fujitsu.com/global/news/publications/periodicals/fstj/archives/vol41-1.html

Hosoyama M (2004) The author in conversation with Masakuza Hosoyama, Design Planning Group, Matsushita Electrical Industrial Co Ltd., Tokyo, Japan

IAUD (2005) Bulletin 1, International Association for Universal Design, Kanagawa, Japan

JIPRI (2000) Study on universal design. Japanese Industrial Policy Research Institute, Quoted in AXIS 115: 2005, 6, 26, AXIS, Tokyo, Japan

Macdonald AS (2005) Universal design meets the modern journey: individuals in complex environments. Gerontechnology 3(4): 213

Matsushita (2004) The Panasonic report for sustainability. Matsushita Electric Group

Ohshima M (2004) The author in conversation with Makoto Ohshima, General Manager of the Toyota Raum design team and colleagues, Toyota-shi

Toshiba (2004) Tomorrow's ideas today: Toshiba's universal design. Toshiba Corporation Design Center. Available at: http://toyota.jp/sp/porte/main.html and http://www.city.kyoto.jp/hokenfukushi/hofukusoumu/ud

Chapter 3

Encouraging Inclusive Design Through Standardisation

D.E. Hughes, G. Cockerham and J.S. Paul

3.1 Fit for Inclusion?

The positive benefits of physical activity in health and disease prevention are longstanding and well documented (DoH, 1995). The World Health Organisation (WHO, 2003) identifies lack of physical activity as a major underlying cause of death, disease and disability and as such encourages governments to provide access to play and sporting facilities to improve health. The UK Government's latest strategy (DCMS, 2002) promotes physical activity as a way to gain significant health benefits while concurrently reducing the growing healthcare costs of an increasingly sedentary and ageing population. The circa £3billion UK health and fitness industry (Key Note Ltd., 2002) has directly benefited from these health promotion drives with the implementation of GP referral schemes and initiatives to combat obesity and other health conditions. To cover the diversity of the UK population there is evidently a real need to ensure that physical activity is accessible to all.

3.1.1 The Inclusive Fitness Initiative – Actively Promoting Inclusion

Since its launch in 2001 the Inclusive Fitness Initiative (IFI), delivered under the auspices of the English Federation of Disability Sport, has received £6million of Sport England Lottery funding directed towards removing barriers to participation in fitness faced by disabled people. The IFI works throughout England, in partnership with local authorities and not-for-profit organisations, in the key areas of training, marketing, sports development and equipment provision. Notably the IFI grant aids equipment purchases for existing gym refits and new build sites. By the end of 2005 the IFI will support 180 public sites and also be piloting several private sector sites.

3.1.2 Membership of an Exclusive Fitness Club?

Early work (GJSF, 1999) by the IFI explored attitudes and approaches to disability apparent in the UK fitness industry. The IFI concluded that disabled people were severely under-represented within the industry's estimated 5.8million public and private health and fitness club members (The Leisure Database Company, 2003). Focusing specifically on equipment provision the IFI uncovered a lack of availability, awareness and investment in accessible equipment. Fitness provision for disabled people was largely based on physiotherapy or specialist rehabilitation equipment which rarely featured in mainstream gyms. Other researchers similarly reported that 96% of private facility managers responding to their study stated they did not have equipment suitable for use by disabled users (Access4fitness, 2001). This overwhelming lack of equipment was regarded as a barrier to both existing and new participation in fitness.

3.1.3 Tackling the Issue – IFI Research and Research and Development Associates

Approaches by the IFI to the fitness industry confirmed that fitness equipment had previously received little attention from the inclusive design community. Appropriate resources on inclusive design were scant and dispersed across numerous disciplines and sources. The proactive response to this situation was the formation of a collaborative research development (R&D) project funded by 13 fitness equipment manufacturers, the IFI, Montgomery Leisure Services, Sport England and Sheffield Hallam University. The suppliers group represents a large percentage of the UK market, including many major multinational players along with small and medium sized organisations.

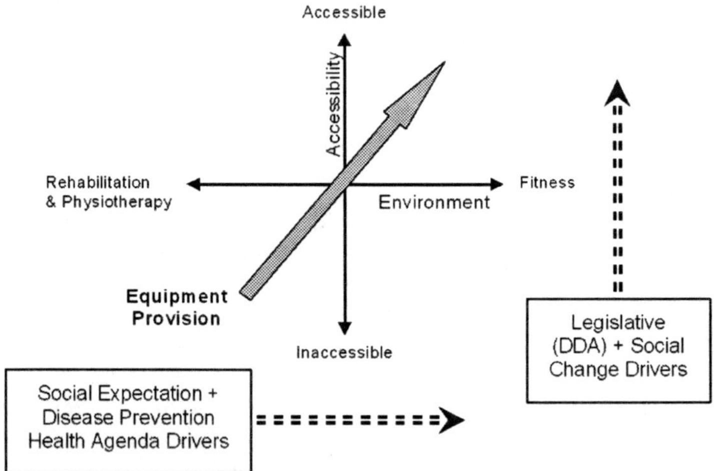

Figure 3.1. Fitness industry transition towards accessible mainstream equipment

The research project undertook to provide practical industrial support to help suppliers understand and meet the needs of disabled people. The principal requirements for the successful design of accessible fitness equipment would be identified and embodied in an inclusive design standard for the industry. Problems with practical implementation of barrier-free equipment design would be tackled to support the industry transition towards truly accessible mainstream equipment production (as illustrated in Figure 3.1).

Rationales cited by suppliers for involvement in the research included commercial gains from increased equipment sales, a positive company profile from a public commitment to inclusion, avoidance of possible litigation against Disability Discrimination Act (1995) requirements and the opportunity to influence future fitness industry standards for accessible design.

3.2 Why Standardise Diversity?

Keates and Clarkson (2003) report that legislation and regulation are amongst the most effective tools for persuading companies to adopt universal design. Although legislation and directives could be used as drivers the IFI perceived that the need was to change the image of inclusive design into something which had credibility in current mainstream corporate culture. In this respect standards would be used as a carrot and not a stick in the largely unregulated fitness industry. The achievement of a recognised standard also facilitated marketing power, which was a particularly attractive element for suppliers. Ultimately this illustrated a commercial incentive and allowed relatively small sales or design teams to have influence and gain support and resources within their organisations.

Communication within supplier organisations emerged as a paramount issue to be considered when developing design standards. In addition to providing a commonality of language for all involved, documented design standards proved invaluable in allowing UK based organisations to communicate effectively with their overseas design departments. The standards documentation embodies a specification for good inclusive product design. Suppliers who outsource their detailed design work to freelance designers or design consultancies utilise the standards as part of their formal product specification to these organisations. As a fixed metric the standards can then be employed throughout the design process to aid decision-making and as a measure of success in final testing and evaluation.

For designers tasked with implementing the standards the imperative was to produce documentation which allowed practical implementation of inclusive design theory in a commercial setting, whilst avoiding information overload. Knowledge and communication gaps within the industry were identified as depicted in Figure 3.2 (based on Keates and Clarkson, 2003). Bridging these gaps within a design standard would free designers to focus on creative and resourceful problem solving as opposed to taking on the role of researcher. Consolidation of relevant information would allow designers to be comfortable and competent to problem solve within commercial timeframe and resource constraints.

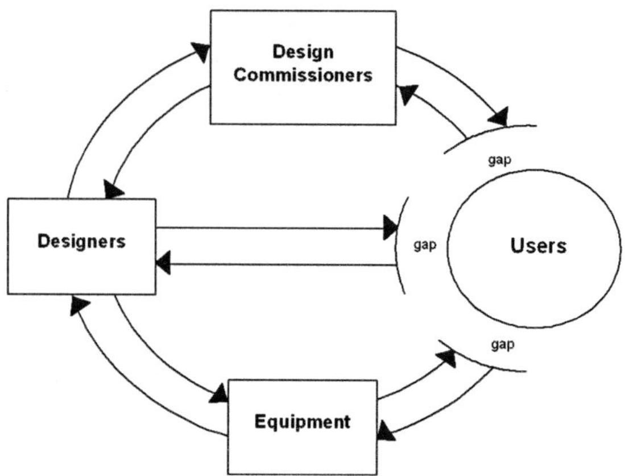

Figure 3.2 Communication and knowledge gap model for the fitness industry

Whilst it is acknowledged that this form of design assistance can support the achievement of inclusive design, the dangers of blindly implementing a design standard without sufficient understanding and appreciation of its essence are also recognised. The authors are keen to stress that provision of a design standard must not be a standalone activity. Standards provision does not negate the need for inclusive design training and support of design teams with standards interpretation and implementation. Additional design educational materials must be provided to encourage and inspire designers to go beyond the minimum accepted level of standards compliance.

Regrettably the removal of direct engagement of designers with disabled users during the design process is a major limitation to the exclusive use of design standards. Consequential effects of user-designer interaction, such as the removal of the fear of engaging with disabled people and spontaneous product innovation/inspiration, are lost. It is therefore essential that designers are encouraged to implement inclusive design standards alongside other user-centred design practices. Use of both consultants and expert users has been reported from within the fitness industry. These experiences support the process of designer awareness raising, and education and skills development.

Although the standards development process has proved a successful awareness raising exercise both within the fitness industry and with disabled people involved in the development process, this is seen as a short term benefit. To provide for long term sustainability of inclusive design within the fitness industry the IFI has targeted the integration of their design standard within BS EN 957 – the British and European safety standard for fitness equipment (BSI, 1997). The forthcoming update of BS EN 957 will incorporate a new "inclusive use" classification for which the IFI design standards are referenced in the bibliography as the only nationally recognised guidance document. To further embed inclusion within the fitness industry, the IFI has successfully penetrated local authority procurement processes, effectively making it difficult for new equipment not meeting the IFI standards to be purchased.

With the IFI design standards increasingly entering the public domain the need for them to be formalised and well documented becomes vital. The standards allow for a transparent and validated process of equipment development and assessment to be maintained. Working within a large commercial group, confidentiality and fairness issues frequently prevailed. Generic and consistent presentation of information, inherent in formatting standards, was essential to ensure fairness and equity. In this way the IFI has been able to retain influence and co-operation with the fitness industry as a whole, ensuring the widespread commercial availability of accessible products in the UK market.

3.3 Approaching Standardisation

3.3.1 Capturing User Needs

Following a 'countering design exclusion' approach (Keates and Clarkson, 2003) the first stage in the development of design standards was identification of barriers to current equipment usage. This warranted a data collection methodology that would allow formalisation and codification of tacit knowledge from disabled users whilst ensuring their voices remained at the centre of any research and assessment procedures. A technique based on practical interaction with equipment was used to capture user wants, needs and aspirations for equipment development.

Feedback of user satisfaction with current equipment was collected at five commercially based research days (accreditation sessions) held over a three year period. Questionnaires utilised a six point (0-5) scale to investigate design issues of ease of access/egress, adjustability, ease of use/programming, range of movement, range of resistance and comfort. Qualitative feedback was solicited to support qualitative scores. These pan-disability sessions, with testers self-declaring impairment, included non-disabled testers and focused on disability as opposed to ageing. The resulting data set comprised opinions from 127 testers on over 200 individual pieces of commercial fitness equipment. Key findings from the test sessions identified a lack of equipment provision for those with sensory impairments and learning disabilities. Users with asymmetric strength or limited dexterity were also poorly catered for. Data collection methodologies and detailed findings are described in Paul and Hughes (2004) and Hughes *et al.* (2005).

3.3.2 A Staged Approach to Industrial Change

Presenting designers solely with the raw user test session data was considered of limited usefulness due to the volume of data collected. Therefore the essential findings were described and published as an initial set of design standards (IFI, 2004). These 'stage one' standards lacked detailed quantitative design information in some areas due to voids in knowledge about exact user requirements and the most effective ways of satisfying these needs. Also omitted were areas for which long supplier lead-in times were required.

Reinforcing the iterative nature of standards development, the stage one standards did however prove crucial in forming a basis document from which further specific research areas could be identified. The areas prioritised for further research were driven by industrial knowledge gaps and a focus on those users identified as being most excluded by current equipment designs. Notably, clear and easy access to equipment, ease of use of adjustments (particularly for unilateral use), simplicity of programming and use of multi-sensory information on user-product interfaces (audio feedback, tactile labelling and effective use of colour) were targeted for further investigation. Increasingly specific user testing was employed to address the need for greater clarity and quantification of user requirements in these areas.

Thirty individual test scenarios were established and tests conducted to elicit more equipment and component specific information for direct integration into the standards documentation. Test questionnaires gave a focus for testers to consider and compare individual product components and state their preferences when presented with multiple options for achieving the same equipment outcome.

For these studies tester selection was prescribed and explicit. Importantly testers were selected by specification of functional requirements as opposed to impairment, analogous to the concepts of lead and critical users defined by Von Hippel (1986) and Keates and Clarkson (2003) respectively. Additionally, testers with maximum experience of product use and evaluation were selected alongside a small number of 'new-to-product' testers.

3.3.3 Formalisation of the Standards Development Process

Significant findings from the second round of testing were incorporated as appropriate into the existing standards documentation. This documentation then went through the formal standards development process identified in Figure 3.3. This process closely resembles those formally described by established standards development bodies (ISO, 2003). The decision was taken early to base the format and structure of the IFI standards on that of BS EN 957, as this was a familiar standard to the fitness industry and IFI alike. The structure of the standards is therefore based on presenting a generic Part 1 followed by a number of equipment specific Parts (*e.g.* treadmills, cycles, *etc.*).

3.4 Industrial Perspectives and Supplier Input

Supplier input into the design standards was sought directly at 6 formal R&D forums attended by individual product designers, production managers, sales staff and IFI representatives. Further qualitative and anecdotal information was gathered informally from observational analysis at these forums along with industry press and freeform interviews conducted during site visits and pre- and post-visit telephone and email dialogue. Importantly, a formal supplier consultation period was allocated within the formal standards development process (see Figure 3.3).

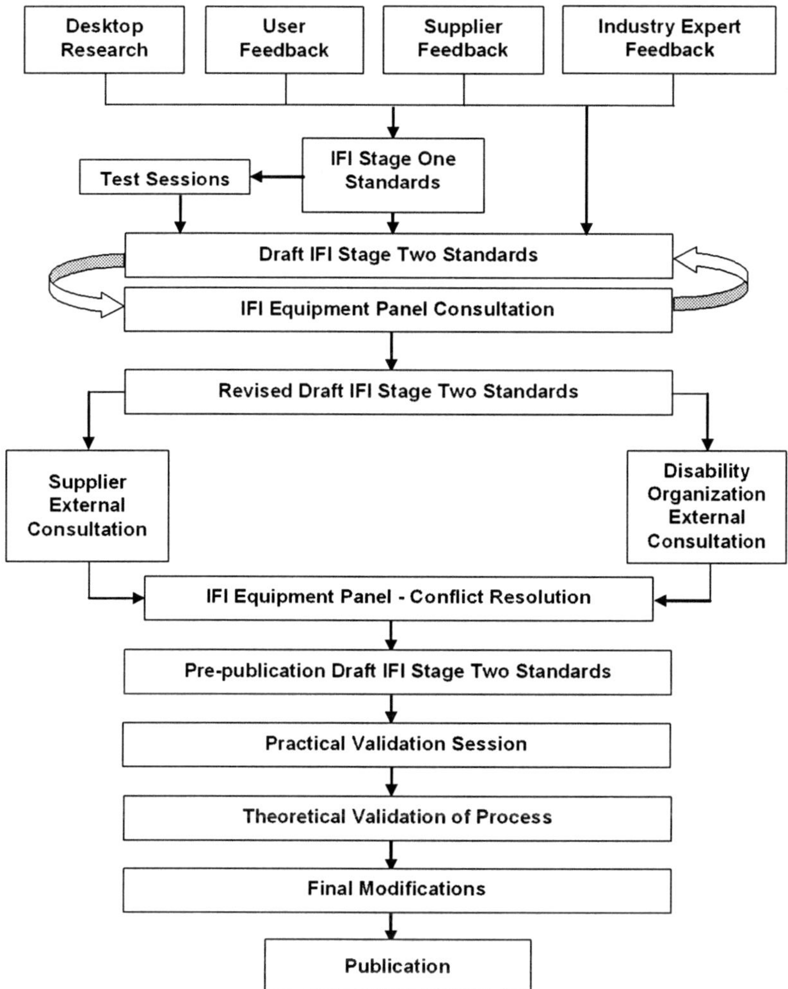

Figure 3.3. Model of the IFI design standards development process

Early supplier feedback concerned commercial imperatives and barriers to adoption of inclusive design rather than specific technical contributions to the standard (Paul and Hughes, 2004). Subsequently however as their knowledge increased, suppliers were able to adopt a more proactive role and input constructively into the details of the standard. Encouraging negotiation and input into the standards documentation by suppliers was seen as essential to securing publication of meaningful and achievable standards, maximising the likelihood of their being adopted and complied with.

3.5 A Balancing Act – The Equipment Expert Panel

For the IFI, successful inclusive design standards would be user-led, with real user needs captured through test sessions, mixed with an injection of commercial reality from supplier feedback. The challenge of balancing these often incongruent requirements was undertaken by the IFI Equipment Panel which comprised industry experts in the fields of fitness equipment design, design legislation, fitness instruction, inclusive sports equipment design, disability equity and an elected supplier representative. Assessments, commentary and judgements on the standards were made through discussions at IFI Equipment Panel meetings.

3.5.1 Diversity of Need – Conflict Resolution

Achieving a balance between competing stakeholder needs encompassed resolution of both user-user and supplier-user needs. To fulfil their responsibility to cohesively merge the supplier position with that of the disabled gym user, the IFI Equipment Panel had to implement prioritisation methods. This hierarchy of considerations was topped by user safety and risk assessment concerns including appropriateness of the exercise. Likely practical achievability followed this based on supplier restrictions of cost, market share, resource allocation, production/ manufacturing limitations, ease of change implementation and expected lead-in times. Anticipated level of inclusion was considered in turn utilising user epidemiology and demography as appropriate to make compromise decisions.

The IFI Equipment Panel had to concede to limitations on the definition of 'inclusive' in inclusive design. In setting the standards a user-aware approach prevailed, where success was seen as pushing mainstream product boundaries to accommodate an increased range of user size and shapes along with appropriate multi-sensory information. There remain users for whom adherence to the IFI standards will not produce truly useable equipment. This emphasises the corresponding ethical issue of what *could be* designed versus what *should be* designed. The boundary between equipment performance and the skill of the user is complex. The aim of the sports equipment designer should be to develop equipment which promotes and facilitates performance whilst encouraging positive skill development (Paul, 2005). Fitness equipment should not overcompensate for functional limitations and remove the necessity for skill development.

3.5.2 The Devil is in the Detail

A complex and time-consuming aspect of imparting detailed decisions on the standards was agreeing exact wording and language usage. Definitions and agreed understanding of terminology were vital along with achieving comprehensive coverage of possible design options. Subtle changes in wording could convey emphasis on a different aspect of the standard or change its meaning completely.

Wherever possible the wording of the standard was chosen to allow interpretation and development of novel or unique solutions whilst staying within inclusive design parameters. An additional challenge to standards writing was anticipating and providing coverage about the nature and form of equipment which has yet to be developed!

3.6 Standards Validation

Validation exercises were performed for both the data collection and standards development methodologies. A practical validation session was held to formally assess the ease of application of the standards to current fitness equipment designs. Informal comparisons between the stage one and stage two standards were undertaken. Additionally all primary stakeholders were formally asked to reflect critically on their experiences and this data was combined with pre-standard data to evaluate bias and consistency and provide triangulation of findings. Explorations of parity of the completed standards with other documented inclusive design models and resources are currently being pursued.

3.7 Conclusions

Standards development is an iterative process for which a rational development approach may commence with detection of true user needs and aspirations. Subsequently these needs must be negotiated with relevant industrial partners to achieve appropriate, meaningful and achievable standards. An independent body of experts may facilitate this negotiation and assist with inevitable conflict resolution issues. Successful standards should represent a design brief and specification for achievable product design which ensures the needs of more diverse users are met.

The IFI have been able to effect sustainable change in the UK fitness equipment industry through the development of inclusive design standards. Using this approach the IFI has been able to successfully influence the industry as a whole to achieve practical implementation of inclusive design. In terms of equipment development the IFI has demanded new designs, manufacturing techniques and colour ways from supplier products. Suppliers have encompassed these requirements and their accomplishments are elaborated in Hughes *et al.* (2005). Products widely available in the UK market now lead Europe, the USA and the rest of the world in terms of inclusive commercial fitness equipment design. This represents a real move for inclusive design beyond work, educational and activities of daily living products into pleasurable products to achieve long term health benefits.

3.8 Acknowledgements

The authors would like to thank the IFI accreditation and test day participants, Montgomery Leisure Services staff involved in the IFI and the R&D Associates for their invaluable input and support.

3.9 References

Access4fitness (2001) The access4fitness report: access for disabled people to UK fitness facilities. Available at: http://www.access4fitness.org.uk/

BSI (1997) BS EN 957-1: stationary training equipment – general safety requirements and test methods. British Standards Institution, UK

DCMS (2002) Game plan: a strategy for delivering Government's sport and physical activity objectives. Joint Department of Culture, Media and Sport / Strategy Unit Report – December. UK Cabinet Office, Crown Copyright, UK

DoH (1995) More people, more active, more often. Physical activity in England: a consultation paper. Department of Health, London, UK

Disability Discrimination Act (1995) Available at: http:\\www.disability.gov.uk/legislation

GJSF (Gary Jelen Sports Foundation) (1999) Report on the findings of the national survey into access to fitness facilities for disabled people. English Federation of Disability Sport and Montgomery Leisure Services Ltd., UK

von Hippel E (1986) Lead users: a source of novel product concepts. Management Science 32(7): 791–805

Hughes D, Paul S, Cockerham G (2005) Industrial barriers to practical implementation of inclusive semantics in commercial fitness equipment design. In: Proceedings of INCLUDE 2005, Royal College of Art, London, UK

IFI (2004) Fitness equipment standards stage one. Inclusive Fitness Initiative Equipment Panel, Sheffield Hallam University, UK

ISO (2003) Stages of the development of International Standards. International Organization for Standardisation. Available at: http:\\www.iso.org/iso/en/stdsdevelopment/whowhen how/proc/proc.html

Keates S, Clarkson PJ (2003) Countering design exclusion: an introduction to inclusive design. Springer, London, UK

Key Note Ltd. (2002) Health clubs and leisure centres. March 2002 Market Report

Paul S (2005) Inclusive adventure by design. In: Proceedings of INCLUDE 2005, Royal College of Art, London, UK

Paul S, Hughes D (2004) Embracing human diversity through inclusive design of commercial fitness equipment. The Engineering of Sport 5, International Sports Engineering Association 1: 234–240

The Leisure Database Company (2003) The state of the industry report 2003. Press release. Available at: http:\\www.online-leisure.com/2003pressrelease.html

WHO (2003) Physical activity, sedentary lifestyle: a global public health problem. Non-communicable disease prevention and health promotion. World Health Organization. Available at: http:\\www.who.int/hpr/physactiv/sedintary.lifestyle1.shtml

Chapter 4

Factors Involved in Industry's Response to Inclusive Design

J. Goodman, H. Dong, P.M. Langdon and P.J. Clarkson

4.1 Introduction

In this paper, we present results from an ongoing survey, drawing on responses from 87 UK companies from the design, manufacturing and retail sectors. We examine the factors involved in industry's response to inclusive design, particularly focusing on the drivers and barriers to inclusive design adoption. We ask whether these factors vary according to the company's current situation and whether this can help us to provide inclusive design promotion and support tools that are more suited to the issues faced by different companies.

4.1.1 Motivation

There are great potential benefits to a company from widening its target market to encompass all users, including those who are older or have disabilities. Yet many companies still target young, fit people, both in their own designs and when commissioning and buying products from others. To overcome this hurdle, we need to understand what causes it and gain a more complete picture of the current situation; the reasons that companies themselves give for not designing more inclusively and the things that they feel would encourage them to design more inclusively in the future.

4.1.2 Related Work

Previous studies have identified some of these barriers to and drivers towards inclusive design. In the US, the Universal Design Research Project (UDRP) carried out telephone interviews with 26 US consumer product manufacturers

(Vanderheiden and Madison, 1998; Vanderheiden and Tobias, 2000) and a similar study was conducted with 307 Japanese companies (Unpublished, 2000). Both studies identified a range of barriers and drivers for universal (or inclusive) design, covering areas such as government regulation, training and education, market data, consumer and society demand, technical complexity and (the lack of) interest, knowledge and techniques.

More recently, in the UK, Dong *et al.* (2004) surveyed a range of manufacturers, retailers and design consultancies to identify their perceived drivers and barriers to inclusive design. They describe how the barriers fall into the three main categories of perception, technical and organisational and discuss how these barriers vary from sector to sector.

Results from these studies indicate some of the key barriers and drivers to inclusive design. However, they also show that there are many different kinds of these, varying from company to company. It is important to understand more about this variation so that efforts to overcome barriers and to support drivers can be better suited to the needs of individual companies. The work reported in this paper seeks to increase this understanding by identifying the factors involved in companies' responses to inclusive design and asking whether these factors vary according to the type of company.

4.1.3 Context

The survey described in this paper was created and initiated as part of a project sponsored by the UK Department of Trade and Industry (DTI). This project aimed to raise awareness of the commercial imperative of inclusive design. In particular, it sought to survey industrial awareness of inclusive design and to develop high impact inclusive design training for managers (Goodman *et al.*, 2005). Preliminary results from the survey provided the basis for focusing on the business case in the training package and following this up with practical knowledge and tools.

The work was also carried out as part of the EPSRC funded i~design project, which seeks to better enable industry to design products that can be used effectively by the population as a whole, including those who are older or disabled. The survey supports this project in its provision of practical and effective support to industry by providing an increased understanding of the commercial setting. It forms part of a convergent approach, in which multiple methods are used to investigate designers' work practices, with the aim of providing designers with more effective and suitable guidance and information on inclusive design (Goodman *et al.*, 2006b).

This survey builds on a previous UK study, described above (Dong *et al.*, 2004; Dong, 2004). It seeks to address some of the previous study's limitations by expanding the size of the sample and investigating companies' demographics and current position in more detail.

Some of the results from this survey have been published elsewhere (Goodman *et al.*, 2006). That paper presents general results while the current paper focuses on the factors involved in a company's response to inclusive design and the differences between different types of companies. The survey is on-going (as of autumn 2005) with both papers presenting intermediate results. Although the results are intermediate and so not from the complete final sample, we believe that the sub-sample is sufficiently large to provide interesting and useful information for those seeking to provide guidance and information to designers and to industry on inclusive design.

4.2 Method

4.2.1 Questionnaire Structure

The questionnaire was divided into six main parts: company profile; current understanding (of inclusive design and related concepts); current company position (on inclusive design); drivers for inclusive design; barriers to inclusive design; and approaches to increase the usage of inclusive design.

The first three parts were designed to enable understanding of the context of the response. They sought to understand aspects of this context such as whose point of view the completed questionnaire represented and the company's current situation with respect to inclusive design. At the start of the third part of the questionnaire, the following definition of inclusive design was given: "a process whereby designers, manufacturers and service providers ensure that their products and services address the needs of the widest possible audience, irrespective of age or ability" (derived from the DTI's Foresight Programme). This definition was used to ensure that subsequent responses were given with a common understanding of inclusive design.

Parts 4 and 5 listed major drivers and barriers that were identified in a previous UK survey (Dong *et al.*, 2004). Since the new survey was part of a larger project aimed at raising awareness of the commercial imperative behind inclusive design, drivers that were relevant to the business case were broken down into several more detailed drivers, such as "entrance to a new market", "achieve a larger share of your current market" and "increase customer satisfaction".

For both parts 4 and 5, comment boxes were provided so that other key drivers and barriers could be added. Most of the questions asked for responses on a scale of 1 to 4, so that answers could be ranked. Where this was not the case, *e.g.* in Part 5 (Barriers to inclusive design), where 'Yes' and 'No' answers were collected, further questions were added to obtain ranking data, *e.g.* "of the above barriers, which is the most important?".

The options in Part 6 (Approaches to increase the usage of inclusive design) were designed to fit with the specific foci of the larger DTI project and the insights of the research team, although other tools could be added in the comment box. For example, suggested tools included "Attending a DTI / Design Council Inclusive Design event" and "Receiving an exclusion assessment on your product / service".

4.2.2 Sampling and Questionnaire Distribution

This paper presents intermediate results from an ongoing survey. To date, complete responses have been obtained from 87 UK companies from the design, manufacturing and retail sectors. Several partial responses were also received but are not included in the results reported in this paper. The questionnaire was distributed by a variety of methods. Many of the responses were obtained through industry contacts, while others were recruited by phoning contacts obtained through a web search. A sampling analysis is underway but early results suggest that companies were predominantly sampled from the Midlands, South East and London areas. The sample is essentially self-selected, implying some interest in or knowledge of inclusive design prior to the questionnaire. It seems likely, then, that the sample is generalisable to this geographic and economic area. It is also likely to include a higher proportion of organisations with prior awareness of inclusive design than in the design community as a whole. The analysis in this paper takes this into account by explicitly examining companies' self-reported level of awareness of inclusive design and investigating its effect on other aspects studied in the questionnaire.

4.3 Results

4.3.1 Main Drivers and Barriers for Companies as a Whole

Respondents were asked how much they agreed with a set of statements about drivers for inclusive design. Key drivers for companies as a whole were brand enhancement, and demographic and consumer trends. When they were then asked how effective they thought inclusive design could be in helping them to achieve a range of commercial benefits, respondents highlighted increasing customer satisfaction and providing a source of innovation and differentiation.

Part 5 then asked respondents whether or not they agreed with statements on barriers to inclusive design. The biggest barrier was the lack of time and budget to support it. Other significant barriers were a lack of knowledge and tools to practise it and the feeling that inclusive design was not a perceived need of their end users.

More details on the drivers and barriers chosen, as well as general results of the survey, are given in Goodman *et al.* (2006).

4.3.2 Key Factors in Response to Inclusive Design

A factor analysis was carried out on a subset of 25 questions from the questionnaire to determine the main factors affecting the companies' responses to inclusive design, particularly their responses to possible barriers and drivers to inclusive design. The analysis was conducted in SPSS using Principal Component Analysis with Varimax Kaiser normalised rotation of components. Questions on companies' responses to the barriers and drivers were chosen, along with some questions describing the companies' current situation, particularly in terms of their current response to inclusive design (see Figure 4.1 for details).

A Kaiser-Meyer-Olkin Measure of sampling adequacy indicated good common variance at 0.631 and Bartlett's Test of non-sphericity indicated highly significant relationships between the variables. Rotation of the factor components did not produce a stronger fit over the factors derived. The communalities analysis indicated that all the variables contributed substantially to the final analysis and that a scree plot of eigenvalues indicated a strong change in slope between 4 and 5 factor components.

The analysis was interpreted to establish four key factors over companies' responses as shown in Table 4.1 on the following page and outlined below (note that the descriptions of the factors summarise their elements only roughly):

- Factor 1: awareness of barriers and desire or motivation for change;
- Factor 2: arguments for the commercial value of inclusive design;
- Factor 3: possible effects of inclusive design on company market position;
- Factor 4: resources, skills and tools needed for inclusive design.

4.3.3 Key Factors in Response to Specific Barriers and Drivers

Of particular interest for our purposes is the influence of different variables on companies' responses to the different barriers and drivers for inclusive design. There are many different variables that could be examined but, for an initial analysis, we chose to look at one of the key parts of the first factor identified by the factor analysis, that is, the current level of awareness of inclusive design in an organisation. This is an important factor in itself and is closely coupled with responses to various barriers within Factor 1. Therefore, further analysis investigated the relationship between this variable and the specific barriers and drivers.

Graphs of the barriers identified for different levels of awareness are shown in Figure 4.1 and illustrate the effect of this variable. Increased awareness of inclusive design was related to lower barriers overall, except for the stigma associated with inclusive design (already a low barrier) and, to some extent, the perception that inclusive design compromises the aesthetics of a design.

In general, as shown in Figure 4.2, greater awareness of inclusive design was also associated with a more positive response to all of the key drivers, except for "British Standard BS7000-6 will help us to practice and manage Inclusive Design". Its low effect on this particular driver was probably due to a low awareness of this British Standard among companies in the survey in general.

Table 4.1. Component matrix: Four key factors in companies' responses and their factor loadings. ID is an abbreviation for inclusive design. Where a statement is given, respondents were asked how much they agreed with it for their organisation.

No.	Question (abbreviated)	1	2	3	4	
3.1	Level of awareness of ID	.753				Factor 1
3.2	Current inclusivity of products/services	.676	-.362			Factor 1
5.1a	There is little or no internal support for ID	-.666				Factor 1
5.1d	There is no justifiable business case to support ID	-.663				Factor 1
5.1e	There is a lack of time and budget to support ID	-.606				Factor 1
5.1c	We lack the knowledge and tools to practise ID	-.585	.314	.349		Factor 1
4.2a	ID would help to achieve entrance to a new market	.501	.378			Factor 1
5.1b	ID would require significant cultural change	-.496		.326	-.344	Factor 1
3.5a	Awareness of the DDA (Disability Discrimination Act) or ADA (Americans with Disabilities Act)	.446	-.444		-.389	Factor 1
4.2c	ID would help to achieve more of the current market	.475	.642			Factor 1
3.5b	Awareness of British Standard BS7000-6 (Managing Inclusive Design)	.445				Factor 2
4.2g	ID would produce innovation and differentiation	.403	.621			Factor 2
6.1a	A convincing argument (business case) for top level management is important for encouraging ID		.616			Factor 2
4.1c	Social responsibility is a key driver for ID		-.532			Factor 2
4.3	ID could be effective in enhancing our brand	.418	.504			Factor 2
5.1i	There is a stigma associated with ID			.631		Factor 3
5.1g	ID compromises the aesthetics of the design			.567		Factor 3
4.1d	Demographic/consumer trends are key drivers for ID			.426	-.345	Factor 3
4.1a	Legislation is a key driver for ID		-.307	.362		Factor 3
4.1e	Brand enhancement is a key driver for ID			.457		Factor 3
4.1b	BS7000-6 will help us to practise and manage ID				.609	Factor 4
1.1	Number of employees				-.603	Factor 4
6.1c	Skills or tools to assist with designing inclusively are important for encouraging ID		.333	.408	.495	Factor 4
1.5	Existence of a post for corporate social responsibility				.471	Factor 4
6.1d	Tools to market ID are important for encouraging ID	.327	.414		.467	Factor 4

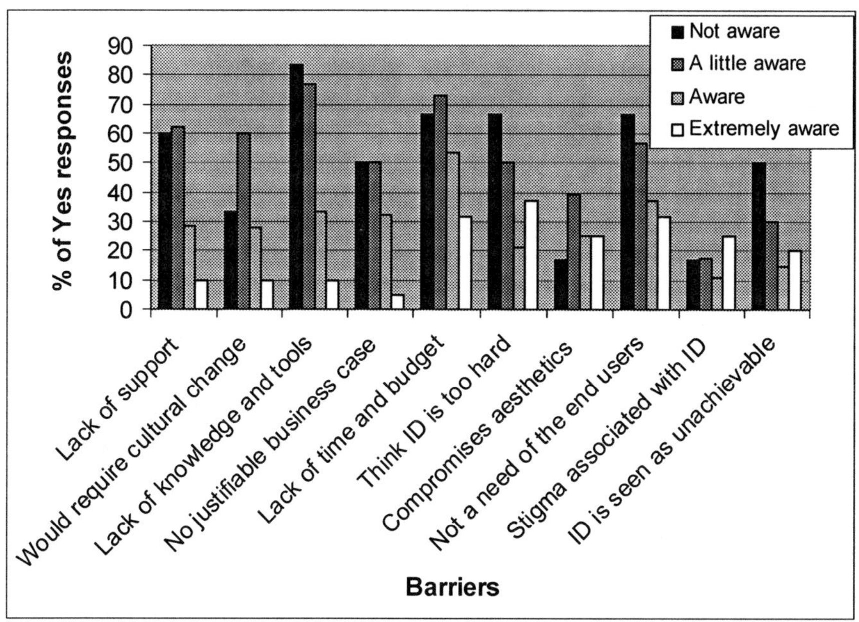

Figure 4.1. Response to suggested barriers to inclusive design for companies with different levels of awareness of inclusive design.

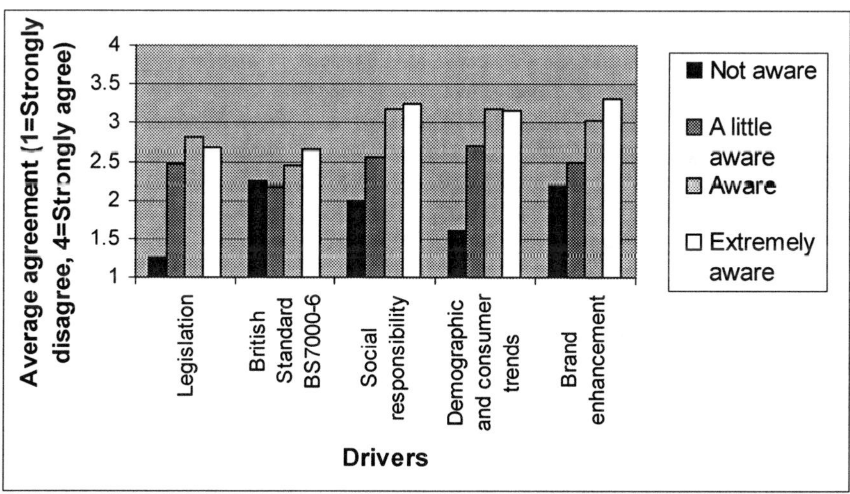

Figure 4.2. Response to suggested drivers for companies with different levels of awareness of inclusive design. Agreement with a driver was rated on a scale of 1 to 4.

4.3.4 More about Current Company Position

The factor analysis examined two of the variables describing current company position: the level of awareness of inclusive design and how inclusive the company thought its products or services currently were. These variables grouped together within a single factor (Factor 1) but closer inspection shows that they relate to each other and to the other current company position variables (the level of effort invested in inclusive design and the level of interest in making products and services more inclusive) in a non-trivial manner. There are some distinct categories of responses, such as companies with a high level of awareness, effort, interest and current inclusivity; a high level of awareness and effort but low inclusivity in practice; high awareness and inclusivity but low interest in improving it; and low levels of awareness.

The previous section showed that the level of awareness of inclusive design has an effect on the response to barriers and drivers and we hypothesise that the other company position variables will also have an effect. Further, we hypothesise that companies falling into different categories with respect to company position, as described above, will have different responses to barriers and drivers. Once the full data set has been obtained, we plan to carry out a fuller factor analysis, including these variables, and also to study these categories in more detail.

4.4 Conclusions and Future Work

For inclusive design to be put into practice successfully we must equip designers, retailers and manufacturers to overcome the barriers to inclusive design and we need to enable and support those aspects that encourage and drive companies to take it up. However, not all companies face the same barriers and drivers. Depending on their current situation with respect to inclusive design, there are different drivers that need to be emphasised and different barriers to be overcome. In practice, this means that different support and training materials and tools need to be developed depending on the companies' current position.

This paper has presented some initial results, starting to identify how companies differ and what their differing needs are but work is needed to explore these differences in more detail. We plan to continue the survey described in this paper, to obtain a larger sample, producing more significant results. In particular, we plan to examine whether companies fitting different patterns as to their current situation have different responses to inclusive design.

We are also continuing work on developing methods to overcome the barriers and aid the drivers identified through the survey. The survey was initially part of a project sponsored by the DTI, which produced a high impact training package to introduce executives to inclusive design. This work is being followed up by the Centre for Inclusive Technology and Design (CITD), in particular by developing a three-day training workshop, equipping designers to put inclusive design into practice.

4.6 References

Dong H, Clarkson PJ, Keates S (2004) Requirements capture for inclusive design resources and tools. In: Proceedings of ESDA 2004, Manchester, UK

Dong H (2004) Barriers to inclusive design in the UK. PhD-thesis, Engineering Department, University of Cambridge, UK

Goodman J, Clarkson PJ, Langdon PM (2005) Developing tools for communicating inclusive design principles. In: Proceedings of a workshop at ADDW 2005, Dundee, UK

Goodman J, Dong H, Langdon PM, Clarkson PJ (2006) Industry's response to inclusive design: a survey of current awareness and perceptions. In: Proceedings of Ergonomics 2006, Cambridge, UK

Goodman J, Langdon PM, Clarkson PJ (2006b) Providing strategic user information for designers: methods and initial findings. In: Clarkson PJ *et al.* (eds.) Designing accessible technology. Springer, London, UK

Unpublished report (2000) Kyoyo-hin (universal design) in Japan. Available from the i~design collection of the Helen Hamlyn Research Centre, Royal College of Art, UK

Vanderheiden G, Tobias J (2000) Universal design of consumer products: current industry practice and perceptions. Available at: http://trace.wisc.edu/docs/ud_consumer_products _hfes2000/ index.htm

Vanderheiden G, Madison J (1998) Barriers, incentives and facilitators for adoption of universal design practices by consumer product manufacturers. Available at: http://www.tracecenter.org /docs/hfes98_barriers/barriers_incentives_facilitators.htm

Chapter 5

Providing Strategic User Information for Designers: Methods and Initial Findings

J. Goodman, P.M. Langdon and P.J. Clarkson

5.1 Introduction

This paper reports initial findings from part of the EPSRC funded i~design project, addressing the usability of user data during the inclusive design process. In order to provide useful user information, it is important to understand how designers work and how they use such information. We, therefore, report a set of findings from a literature review on this topic and describe how this review fits into a longer-term integrated methodology, as a first stage in a convergent approach. We describe the context and role of this work in the overall project and illustrate how the questions and considerations that were yielded by the literature review will act as input to the next observational stage. In addition, we consider the implications of these initial findings for communicating with designers.

5.1.1 Background

There is an increasing acknowledgement of the importance of making designs accessible to the wider population including older and disabled people. The ageing population in developed countries, such as the UK, means that this is a large and increasing group (U.S. Census Bureau, 2005) and one with considerable spending power (Coleman, 2001). In addition, legislation such as the Disability Discrimination Act (DDA) in the UK requires companies to consider the needs of these user groups because both older and disabled groups are disadvantaged and hampered in their use of everyday products due to functional demands beyond their capabilities (Keates and Clarkson, 2003). There is, therefore, clearly a drive to develop more inclusive design solutions (Yelding, 2003) that address users' wants and needs during the design process. However, companies and their designers do not always know how to meet these needs. There is a lack of clarity about the characteristics of the user population, and a lack of knowledge about how to address these in design. If there are going to be truly accessible and usable products in the marketplace, it is imperative to provide companies and designers with more information and guidance on inclusive design.

In order to provide information and guidance that are really usable to the product designer it is necessary to establish the nature, timing and value of the diverse forms of information that are required. In particular, it is unclear what balance is required between methods of obtaining user data that involve direct observation of users such as focus groups, and those that provide data about users such as statistics, introspection and expert audit. Appropriate information and guidance needs to be tailored to designers' work contexts, practices and ways of working. We need to understand what information and methods designers currently use, what characteristics aid in their adoption, and which methods fit well or badly with their work practices (Goodman *et al.*, 2005).

5.1.2 Context

The i~design project, funded by the UK Engineering and Physical Sciences Research Council (EPSRC), seeks to better enable industry to design products that can be used effectively by the population as a whole, including those who are older or disabled. This project focuses on how to put inclusive design into practice in a commercial setting, aiming to merge separate tools and techniques into an integrated holistic approach and to bridge the gaps in the flow of information about users, identified in earlier work on the tools and techniques of inclusive design (Keates and Clarkson, 2003) (see Figure 5.1).

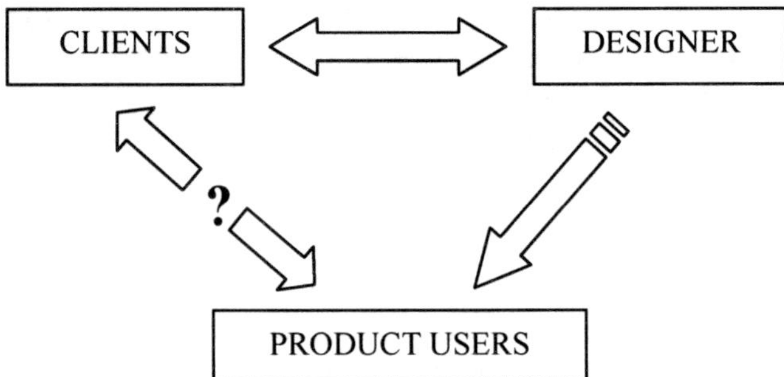

Figure 5.1. Clients talk to designers but there is little communication with users

The current phase of the research aims to investigate the balance between involving users and using data in the design process. An essential element of this is a deeper understanding of designers' work practices including the methods they currently use to inform design and those they would be open to in terms of cost, resources and existing practices. The final objective is to develop a framework for guidance during the design process, in particular for guidance on the choice of methods of acquiring user data and the usefulness and accuracy of the result for differing stages of the design process.

5.2 Methodology

In this paper, we present the first stage of our investigation, part of an approach using a convergent methodology. In this approach, we use a number of research methods that are, in principle, capable of independent results, to address the same set of research questions. Each method has its own advantages and disadvantages with respect to objectivity, accuracy and the degree to which it is capable of revealing unobvious features of designers' work practices. Using a convergent approach allows findings to be cross-checked against each other, avoids favouring any one interpretation, helps to balance the disadvantages of the particular methods, benefits from their advantages and obtains a spectrum of views at different levels of objectivity (Langdon *et al.*, 2003).

The particular methods used are shown in Figure 5.2. It is expected that insights from the literature, survey data, interpreted observational data and recorded retrospective interviews with experts can be used together to obtain a rounded picture of design practice and so inform the development of guidance and methods for designers. We have currently carried out the literature review and are conducting the survey and observational studies.

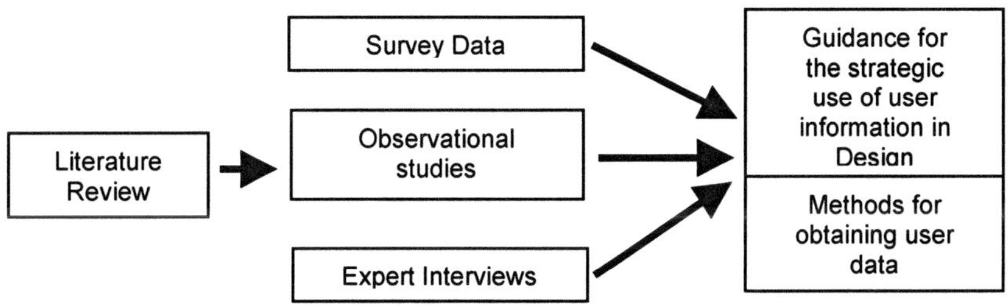

Figure 5.2. The convergent approach to project methodology

5.2.1 Literature Review

As a first step, we have carried out a review of the diverse literature on designers' work practices, from fields such as HCI, engineering design, product design, social science, methodology and psychology. As well as the published literature, we have drawn on raw data from studies carried out on parallel projects (Crilly, 2005; Lebbon, 2005). A summary of the findings is given in Section 5.3.

5.2.2 Observational Study

Using findings from the literature review and earlier projects to define structured questions, we are conducting an observation and interview study of the six design teams involved in the 2005 Design Business Association (DBA) Design Challenge

(DBA, 2005). This is an annual competition, organised by the DBA in association with the Royal College of Art, challenging teams to work with disabled users over a period of about six months, to create examples of inclusive design. Three of this year's teams lie in product design and three in communication design.

Audio and visual data is being collected through observing these teams' design process in formal meetings and interactions with users. We particularly focus on teams' interactions with disabled users, the information used and how this affects the design process. Three of the teams are investigated in more detail. They were selected to represent both product and information design and to spread previous experience of the DBA challenge through employee migration. These teams are being tracked in detail, with semi-structured interviews on their design processes and methods and further observations of team meetings. Informal and workday team member interactions when researchers are not present are captured using retrospective interviews, audio diaries and phone interviews. This challenge presents a unique opportunity to track the processes of three different companies from start to finish of a design, within a manageable time-span, as well as to observe the effect of interaction with disabled users upon this process. This also allows the possibility of examining the relationship between company type, experience and background and the use of design data.

5.2.3 Surveys

To complement this detailed data on designers' behaviour, we are currently conducting a survey into awareness of, barriers to and motivations for inclusive design in companies across the design, retail and manufacturing sectors in the UK. This should yield a more generalisable quantitative statistical perspective on design companies' attitudes towards inclusivity in the design process. The information from this survey will also be backed up with data from a small-scale survey carried out earlier in the i~design project (Lebbon, 2005). Preliminary results from the survey can be found in (Goodman *et al.*, 2006a, 2006b).

5.2.4 Expert Interviews

To complement the survey, literature and observational data and to facilitate the comparison of findings, detailed interviews will be carried out with an expert DBA challenge facilitator, who has selected, briefed and assisted company teams during the challenge for six years. Her role, in particular, has been to introduce teams to the use of observational user data during critical user forums, about midway through the challenge period. This involves exposing the teams to users of products and encouraging them to engage with the lives and capability limitations of these "disabled" forum volunteers in their specific design area (Dong *et al.*, 2005).

5.2.5 Convergent Methodology

The weaknesses of these various methods will be taken into account when comparing and contrasting their outputs. These weaknesses include the unrepresentative nature of the DBA challenge; effects of knowledge of recording during observations; and possible interpretation biases during data segmentation and analysis. Likewise we expect sampling bias, statistical non-representativeness and self-selection biases to affect the survey data. The expert interviews will reflect the participants' biases and weaknesses of memory as well as revealing key insights. The use of a convergent methodology allows an analysis of common findings, the elimination of artefacts resulting from the weaknesses of specific methods and the recording of a spectrum of views at different levels of objectivity.

5.3 Literature Review: Abbreviated Results

This section reports results from the literature review, the first stage of the convergent approach, as described above. These results identify key research themes and specific issues, which will be addressed in the later stages of the investigation.

5.3.1 The Design Process

It is common for descriptions of both the engineering and product design processes in the literature to divide them into a series of stages or phases. While there are some arguments against such a division (Baxter, 1995), the general consensus seems to be that this does indeed describe important aspects of the design process, despite evidence for non-linearity and iterative sub-processes (see Section 3.1.2).

5.3.1.1 Main Phases of Design

Many different design phases are suggested in the literature. However, many of these are similar and can be categorised roughly into six stages, ordered as follows: briefing/defining the problem or opportunity; analysis/data collection; creativity/synthesis; development/prototyping; evaluation/testing; and manufacturing.

How these occur in practice can be illustrated by typical findings. Powell (2005), for example, describes the following design stages: Briefing; Research into social, economic and technological context to establish market relevance; Strategic enquiry and orientation; Idea generation and innovation; Concept design; Concept development; Design development; Further phases and liaison. This illustrates how specific descriptions of the design process fit broadly into the above categories but not in a strict or prescriptive way.

5.3.1.2 Characteristics of the Design Process

In addition, design is not always carried out in the strict linear sequence the above description might suggest. Rather it tends to be iterative, cycling repeatedly through some of the phases and back-tracking to earlier phases (Budgen, 1994). It can also jump around between phases in a less ordered fashion (Restrepo and Christiaans, 2003). What is more, different companies and designers have individualised approaches to design (Lebbon, 2003), though they often still fit into the general, broad set of stages described above (Choueiri, 2003). As well as this, the design process is characterised by a high use of creativity (often specific moments of creativity) (Choueiri, 2003), intuition (Bruseberg and McDonagh-Philp, 2002) and prior experience (Restrepo, 2004).

5.3.2 Design Methods

5.3.2.1 General Design Methods

The literature suggests that a wide range of methods is used in design but that these are not always applied in their formal, accepted form and may be adapted (Bruseberg and McDonagh-Philp, 2002), overlapped and combined according to need. Common design methods, especially in the product design field, include drawing, sketching and modelling (Lawson, 1997; Restrepo, 2004), scenarios (Hasdoğan, 1996) and a variety of subjective and informal techniques, such as the use of previous experience, general guidelines and rules of thumb (Cross, 2000), as well as unfocused browsing (Mival *et al.*, 2004).

5.3.2.2 User Research Methods

Of particular interest for inclusive design are user research practices and methods. There is some variation between disciplines but, again, implicit, subjective techniques dominate, *i.e.* methods such as self-observation, intuition, referring to self-experience or other specialists, looking at related products and obtaining feedback from family and friends (Kotro and Pantzar, 2002).

When more formal methods are used, many designers use the same few methods again and again, whether or not they are appropriate (Cardoso *et al.*, 2005). Particularly common methods early in the design process are questionnaires, interviews and focus groups (Anschuetz, 1996). Later, prototype testing, user trials and checking guidelines are popular (Sims, 2003).

5.3.2.3 Characteristics of Methods

Methods that are commonly used tend to be those that can be adjusted to individual needs and "used in an intuitive and iterative manner" (Bruseberg and McDonagh-Philp, 2002), supporting an informal approach. Also popular are methods that enable designers to visualise their ideas, *e.g.* sketching and modelling. When more formal methods are used, designers seem to prefer a small set of familiar methods. It is also important that methods are suitable for and provide an appropriate level of detail for the current phase of design (Baxter, 1995).

5.3.2.4 Problems with Methods

Various problems with current methods limit their popularity and usefulness. Some formal methods are seen as too "artificial", while others require too many resources, such as time, money, staff and expertise or fit poorly with designers' work practices. In addition, designers can be wary of user research in general, afraid that it will constrain their designing, uncertain of its benefits and resistant to change (Bruseberg and McDonagh-Philp, 2002). Other problems arise, not because of the methods themselves but because of designers' poor understanding of them. A lack of documented reliability and validity, and of information on their strengths and weaknesses can make designers wary of using some methods (Cardello, 2005). When they do use them, the methods are not always applied appropriately or consistently and are often applied in inappropriate situations, leading to "disappointing results and mistrust of methods in general" (López-Mesa and Thompson, 2003).

5.3.3 Information Use

Designers use information in an opportunistic fashion, to complete or confirm facts, to stimulate creativity and occasionally to meet a lack of knowledge (Restrepo, 2004). In addition to that obtained from their own research, formal information about users often comes from sources such as the client (Sims, 2003), a marketing or research department (Hasdoğan, 1996) and published paper and electronic documents (Powell, 1987).

5.3.3.1 Information Formats

Information formats that are commonly used tend to be those that are flexible, familiar and accessible, such as people, paper and product examples. People, especially colleagues and experts, are referred to because they can translate their knowledge to fit designers' requirements (Restrepo and Christiaans, 2003) and because consulting them is "quick and dirty" and can provide a wide range of different kinds of information and build empathy (Cassim, 2005). In engineering design, 24% of a designer's working day was engaged in the acquisition or provision of information and on 90% of these occasions they obtained the information through reference to their colleagues (Marsh, 1997). A comparative study of the outcomes of the US Universal Design Research Project (UDRP) (Vanderheiden, 1998) and the UK Design Business Association (DBA) Design challenge (Cassim, 2005) identified commonalities of findings that included the need for the development of design tools and the generation of statistical and market data for easy reference (Dong *et al.*, 2004).

Paper, in the form of trade and product literature, is used because it is considered reputable, in a format useful for design (Powell, 1987), easily accessible and up-to-date (Rhodes, 1998). Product examples and case studies are also considered to be easy to understand, to use designers' "language" and to be inspirational, enabling one to get an impression of styles, trends and techniques (Rhodes, 1998). Visual formats are better than ones heavy on text, particularly in more creative industries, such as product design, which attract significant proportions of people with dyslexia (Cassim, 2005). Melican found that designers like to form their own concepts of users. They need information that is easy to use and allows them to frame the user interaction in their own way. Both quantitative and qualitative information can be useful for design (Melican, 2000).

5.3.3.2 Problems with Information

Sometimes information supplied to designers is not used. Designers may not use information because they themselves have poor or incorrect representations of the design problem and lack awareness of what information there is or why they need it. They can have a tendency to rely on previous knowledge instead of seeking new information. They may be unwilling to use the information or to change their ideas, and may be unable to transfer the information to their designs. (Powell, 1987; Restrepo, 2004). Some information, however, is not used because of problems with its content or presentation. Common difficulties with its content include poor quality, an unfamiliar and untrusted source and perceived irrelevance (Restrepo, 2004). Another common problem is that the information simply suffers from poor accessibility, *e.g.* it has a poor format or is too text-based (Restrepo and Christiaans, 2003). It may be presented at the wrong level of detail (Restrepo, 2004), be too academic (Morris *et al.*, 2004), too filtered (Crilly, 2005) or buried in other information. It can also come across as too authoritarian (Morris *et al.*, 2004), be hard to get hold of or cost too much (Restrepo, 2004).

5.4 Communicating with Designers

5.4.1 Implications of the Design Process

The design process contains several phases with different characteristics and information needs and it is important to ensure that appropriate methods and information are available for each phase, providing an appropriate level of detail. It is useful to explain what phases each method or piece of information is suitable for, describing the phases in a flexible manner, since different companies use and describe them differently. Design is also characterised by a high use of creativity, intuition and prior experience. Given the high value placed on these and people's reluctance to change, it may be best to support these rather than seeking to replace them. Descriptions of inclusive design methods and information should also avoid any unintentional indications that these features are being replaced.

5.4.2 Implications for Design Methods

Design methods are used very flexibly indicating that a method set or "toolkit" should not provide a neat set of defined formal methods but rather methods that can be overlapped, combined and used in flexible ways. It may be better if such a toolkit is small as designers seem to prefer a small set of familiar methods. If a toolkit is large, then it may be worth-while providing ways of selecting smaller sets, personalised to individual designers, companies or design categories.

When considering individual methods, the problems described in Section 5.3.2.4 show the importance of fit with designers' work practices and budgets and of avoiding artificiality, both in the method itself and in its description. It is also good to remember that implicit and informal methods, like previous experience, general guidelines and rules of thumb, are popular. We should consider how we can support and improve these methods as well as provide replacements. Problems with design methods also arise due to designers' poor understanding of them, what they are and how to apply them. It seems that more information and reassurance about user research in general, more information on individual methods in particular and guidance as to their selection would improve their uptake and use.

5.4.3 Implications for Information Provision

The popular information formats described in Section 5.4.3 provide promising avenues for disseminating information. People, paper (*i.e.* trade literature) and product examples are all useful and well-received formats. When it is not possible or suitable to use them, we can consider how we can replicate their advantages in other formats, for example, translating information to fit particular designers' requirements, enabling quick and easy information access to a wide range of information, encouraging empathy, keeping information up-to-date and using designers' language.

5.5 Conclusions and Future Work

This paper has described the initial results of a literature survey on the design process and designers' work practices, considering practical implications for the provision of information and of design methods, particularly for inclusive design. This survey has provided a rich and extensive source of data about designers' work practices and the use of user data. These results will focus subsequent observation and interview stages and may be considered together with these other methods in a convergent methodology to build a reliable picture of what designers do.

5.6 Acknowledgements

This work is funded by EPSRC through the i~design project.

5.7 References

Anschuetz NF (1996) Evaluating ideas and concepts for new consumer products. In: Rosenau Jr. MD *et al.* (eds.) The PDMA handbook of new product development. John Wiley and Sons, New York, USA

Baxter M (1995) Product design. Nelson Thomas, Cheltenham, UK

Bruseberg A, McDonagh-Philp D (2002) Focus groups to support the industrial/product designer: a review based on current literature and designers' feedback. Applied Ergonomics 33(1): 27–38

Budgen D (1994) Software design. Addison-Wesley, Boston, USA

Cardello AV (2005) Terminology, reliability, validity, and subjectivity in the search for the "voice of the consumer". Food Quality and Preference 16(3): 203–205

Cardoso C, Clarkson PJ, Keates S (2005) Can users be excluded from an inclusive design process? In: Proceedings of HCI International 2005, Las Vegas, USA

Choueiri LS (2003) Diagrams of the design process. In: Proceedings of the 5th European Academy of Design Conference, Barcelona, Spain

Coleman R (2001) Designing for our future selves. In: Preiser WFE, Ostroff E (eds.) Universal design handbook, MacGraw-Hill, New York, USA

Crilly N (2005) Product aesthetics: representing designer intent and consumer response. PhD-thesis, Engineering Department, University of Cambridge, UK

Cross N (2000) Engineering design methods: strategies for product design. John Wiley, Chichester, UK

DBA (Design Business Association) (2005) DBA Design Challenge. Available at: http://www.dba.org.uk/awards/challenge.asp

Dong H, Clarkson PJ, Cassim J, Keates S (2005) Critical user forums – an effective user research method for inclusive design. The Design Journal 8(2): 49–59

Dong H, Keates S, Clarkson PJ (2004) Inclusive design in industry: barriers, drivers and the business case. In: Proceedings of the 8th ERCIM Workshop 'User Interface for All', Vienna, Austria

Goodman J, Langdon P, Clarkson PJ (2005) Providing strategic user information to designers. In: Proceedings of HCI and the Older Population, workshop at HCI 2005, Edinburgh, UK

Goodman J, Dong H, Langdon PM, Clarkson PJ (2006a) Industry's response to inclusive design: a survey of current awareness and perceptions. In: Proceedings of Ergonomics 2006, Cambridge, UK

Goodman J, Dong H, Langdon PM, Clarkson PJ (2006b) Factors involved in industry's response to inclusive design. In: Clarkson *et al.* (eds.) Designing accessible technology. Springer, London, UK

Hasdoğan G (1996) The role of user models in product design for assessment of user needs. Design Studies 17(1): 19–33

Keates S, Clarkson PJ (2003) Countering design exclusion: an introduction to inclusive design. Springer, London, UK

Kotro T, Pantzar M (2002) Product development and changing cultural landscapes – is our future in "snowboarding"? Design Issues 18(2): 30–45

Langdon PM, Aurisicchio M, Clarkson PJ, Wallace K (2003) An integrated ethnographic and empirical methodology in a study of knowledge searches in aerospace design. In: Proceedings of ICED'03, Stockholm, Sweden

Lawson B (1997) How designers think: the design process demystified. Architectural Press, Oxford, UK

Lebbon C (2003) I~design – building a toolkit for inclusive designers. In: Proceedings of INCLUDE 2003, Royal College of Art, London

Lebbon C (2005) I~design DBA questionnaire results. Personal Communication

López-Mesa B, Thompson G (2003) Exploring the need for an interactive software tool for the appropriate selection of design methods. In: Proceedings of ICED'03, Stockholm, Sweden

Marsh JR (1997) The capture and utilization of experience in engineering design. PhD-thesis, Engineering Department, University of Cambridge, UK

Mival O, Smyth M, Benyon D (2004) Crossing the chasm: developing and understanding support tools to bridge the research design divide within a leading product design company. In: Proceedings of Design 2004, Dubrovnik, Croatia

Melican JP (2000) Describing user centered designing: how design teams apply user research data in problem solving. Industrial Design, Illinois Institute of Technology, USA

Morris L, Cooper A, Harun R (2004) Creating a space for practising designers to intellectualise; bringing theory to life for designers. In: Proceedings of Futureground: Design Research Society International Conference 2004, Monash University, Melbourne, Australia

Powell JA (1987) Is architectural design a trivial pursuit? Design Studies 8(4): 187–206

Powell D (2005) About: product design. Design Council, London, UK. Available at: http://www.design-council.org.uk/webdav/servlet/XRM?Page/@id=6004&Session/@id=D_6p40Sj7GyETska9JQz61&Section/@id=1535

Restrepo J (2004) Information processing in design. Delft University Press, The Netherlands

Restrepo J, Christiaans H (2003) Problem structuring and information access in design. In: Proceedings of Expertise in Design, Sydney, Australia

Rhodes P (1998) Abundance of information: how do designers use information? In: Proceedings of IDATER98, Loughborough University, UK

Sims R (2003) 'Design for all': methods and data to support designers. PhD-thesis, Loughborough University, UK

U.S. Census Bureau (2005) International Data Base (IDB). Available at: http://www.census.gov/ftp/pub/ipc/www/idbnew.html

Yelding D (2003) Power to the people. In: Clarkson PJ *et al.* (eds.) Inclusive design: design for the whole population. Springer, London, UK

Chapter 6

Design for Inclusion

D.J. Reed and A. Monk

6.1 Introduction

There has always been a tension between universality and specificity in universal design, seen in various guises, but most prominent in the involvement of user-centred design. We suggest a constructive use of this tension by thinking about the design of distributed socio-technical systems and the targeting of the competencies of various users. We draw on a mentality rooted in soft systems methodology in Human Computer Interaction (HCI) and the sociological approach of Science and Technology Studies. In so doing we envisage a complementary take on inclusive design as *design for inclusion* and present precedents for such a take already existent in the discipline.

While allied to a number of disciplines such as HCI, due to its roots in design, inclusive design has largely concerned itself with individual devices or products. Although a relatively new discipline in itself inclusive design has an historical relationship to other related areas such as "Design for All", "Universal Design" and "Universal Usability" (Newell and Gregor, 2000). As with its parent disciplines, inclusive design contains a tension between a motivation for universality and the specificity seen in its relationship to user centred design. One only has to look at recent inclusive design conferences to see the twin DNA of universality and user-centred research (Keates *et al.*, 2004).

The key to understanding User-Centred Design is the aphorism "know your user". Definitions of usability require that the user group and the task that they are doing be specified. In this context, inclusive design is about defining and understanding your target users, then making sure that all of them are catered for and not excluded because of their particular motor or sensory capabilities (see also Newell and Monk, 2006).

This historical relationship has caused some tension manifested in conversations with, and positioning with regard to, areas such as assistive technology (Newell, 2003). Dan Hawthorn in the design of an email system for older people comments that 'while the interface design decisions made … do assist older users, they limit the power of an application to serve younger, more able and more demanding users' and he makes the argument that 'while it is possible to increase accessibility, the most obvious ways of doing this limit the universality of the resulting application' (Hawthorn, 2003). In this way Hawthorn argues against Schneiderman's assertion that 'dumbing down' and 'innovation restriction' (that restrictions are placed on design) are avoidable when developing systems for older people. Other writers are more positive about developing productive relationships between inclusive design and user centred design. Alan Newell, for example, while maintaining that design for all is a very difficult, if not often impossible task' (Newell and Gregor, 2000), offers an 'new paradigm' called 'User Sensitive Inclusive Design' that extends current User Centred Design methodologies (and is also the title of a continuing set of workshops). The possibility of designing for minorities within a framework geared toward universality is inherent in the term 'inclusive' which waters down the design-for-all objective to design for as many as is practicable. Switching Newell's aphorisms, we might say that this emphasises 'accessibility by most' over 'accessibility for all'.

He also famously recommends a new approach to the underlying question of excluded groups by suggesting a formulation of 'ordinary and extra-ordinary human-machine interaction', that includes a recognition of ability and environment that includes everyone. The argument being that supposedly 'able' people are disabled in certain environments – the sighted in a darkened room, the hearing in the noisy bar, and the mobile phone user wearing gloves.

The recent inclusive design conference was entitled *Designing a More Inclusive World* (Keates *et al.*, 2004) and it is in the spirit of this that we present a reformulation of inclusive design as 'design for inclusion'. This is premised upon work on the social and psychological issues and concerns of older people. This approach takes inclusive designs's underlying political motivation of social inclusiveness and applies it to instances of services based upon distributed technological interventions that involve a number of stakeholders to form a socio-technical system. As such it is meant to extend not only the application of inclusive design but also its definition.

6.2 Expanding the Definition

Inclusive design has already been applied to areas that expand and adapt its typically agreed definiton of "The design of mainstream products and/or services that are accessible to, and usable by, as many people as reasonably possible' (http://www.tiresias.org/guidelines/inclusive.htm). At face value this definition leads to a particular take on inclusive design that is (1) rooted in the individual device, whether that be a tin opener or a car (2) looks for functional parity between the single device and a category of users. Outcomes are usually couched in talk of economic viability, untapped markets and the like. Added to demographic data, this language is used to underpin a rhetoric of persuasion for manufacturers and product designers.

Already in the inclusive design literature this definition is being enlarged to include psychological and sociological issues. At times we see an integration of functional sociological and psychological. So for example, in the area of transport management and urban design, Evans (2005) combines physical functioning issues such as the effect of poorly maintained pavements on those with limited mobility with issues such as crime and the fear of crime. Any response necessarily takes on board safety and the perceptions of the older passenger. As such this combination of factors stands as a template for the inclusion of wider issues, such as we favour.

Some authors stress the vital importance of taking on board wider issues. Hirsch and Forlizzi *et al.* (2002), for example, say that 'failure to consider the social, emotional and environmental dimensions of the aging experience results in missed opportunities for new technologies and applications, and poses difficulties for the adoption of potentially useful products'.

Other authors take up broad international issues. Balaram (2001) points up the socio-ecomomic, cultural and political implications of design: 'Design in the economically developing world is beyond an activity that is concerned with formal qualities and superficial aspects aimed at boosting sales. It is a serious activity that is concerned with playing a key role in economic and social development of the people' (section 5.1). In a similar vein other authors turn inclusive design in on itself and reframe it as a sociologically motivated approach. D'Souza (2004) asks whether Universal Design can be construed as a critical theory, in that it addresses wide ranging social issues such as social emancipation and inclusion, the essential values of technology to different people in different situations and cultures, and the nature of power in the relationships between the designers and manufacturers and the people they make things for.

What is clear from this growing literature is that the focus on single devices and functional ability is only one part of the story. With its roots in senior and disablity rights, and its tendency, already seen, to incorporate wider issues, it is natural that the approach looks to a wider literature and alternative methodologies.

6.3 Design for Inclusion

The approach within inclusive design is typically to start from a design problem normally embodied in a particular device. These problems are detailed in terms of the requirements of different groups of people, including the elderly and the disabled, most commonly in terms of their physical impairments, but also sometimes in terms of psychological and social issues. This then informs a particular product focussed starting point and style of enquiry (see Table 6.1).

An alternative way to formulate inclusive design is to start with broad social psychological and physical concerns and issues faced by particular groups (say the elderly) and allow them to inform 'problem spaces'. Only then do we consider responses to these problems and possible products. This leads to design for inclusion.

One advantage of this reformulation is that we are not primarily drawn to single device solutions. While we may well think in terms of individual devices – say some method of helping a person walk – they are already couched in broader concerns about things like social context (where are they wanting to walk, say) and how that device will impact on other issues and concerns felt by the person. We are also drawn to consider various responses beyond the single device level: perhaps a series of devices, or alternatively devices as part of a socio-technical service.

Table 6.1. A table comparing product and concerns focussed approaches

Product focussed on	**Concerns focussed on**
1. Product with usability problems	1. Analysis of social and psychological issues and concerns (including abilities)
2. Analysis of physical abilities (possibly including social and psychological issues)	2. Identification of problem spaces and product suggestions
3. Inclusive design of existing product	3. New design for inclusion

This alternative way to think about inclusive design then is as *design for inclusion.* This formulation foregrounds the social and psychological issues facing older people, and looks to adapt and develop technologies to address them.

6.4 Social and Psychological Issues

As part of the iDesign project at York we have looked to extend the reach of inclusive design by developing a taxonomy of social and psychological issues facing older people. The analytic approach has been literature based with the supplement of a small number of focus groups and interviews with service professionals.

The motivation is to present the information to designers in such a way as to be accessible, usable and productive. To this end we have developed a list of social and psychological categories, created a table based hyperlinked presentation method, and begun the process of populating the resource from the literature and interviews.The following table contains our current list of the high level social and psychological issues and concerns (see Table 6.2).

Each high level issue – what we call a headline issue - has been developed from our reading of the relevant literature. As can be seen by comparing across the table, social issues usually have a personal or psychological correlation. So for example broad structures of social stigma - when particular groups in society such as the disabled are seen to be discriminated against in areas of employment and the like – relate directly to a personal sense of stigma, that may occur at the level of the labelling affect of using a wheelchair. Indeed a productive way to think about the relationships between the social and the psychological is to imagine how the social impacts on, or is manifested in the experiences of, the personal. It would be a useful exercise to deliberately populate the social issues with personal concerns for example. For the moment we have maintained a distinction and not looked to place the social and psychological in a hierarchical relationship.

Table 6.2. Top level issues and concerns

Social issue or concern	Personal issue or concern
Social exclusion	Personal isolation, participation and activity
Social stigma	Psychological stigma
Age discrimination and ageism	Employment
Elder abuse	Personal injury (physical injury; mental stress)
Independent living	Personal independence
Welfare provision	Wealth and poverty
Health provision	Personal health
Care provision	Personal care
Transport (public and private)	Personal mobility
Technological discrimination (*e.g.* the 'digital divide')	Technophobia
Social empowerment	Personal empowerment
Housing provision	Living environment
Prevention of crime	Fear of crime
Social networks and relationships	Social contact

For every headline issue there is an accompanying information table that details the issue or concern and shows the links to other headline issues. To illustrate how this works we will use the issue of social exclusion. Note: this set of headline issues is developing over the period of the work and may change as new headline issues are added and new categories developed; also we do not wish to suggest that such categories are distinct and a natural grouping scheme. These groups of terms are provided as a point of access to designers to a range of complex issues. The categories are a methodological tool for managing access to complexity, but should always open out to an appreciation of complexity. Therefore the dynamic relationships between our imposed categories are maintained through links across the headline issues, as well as to the subordinate information cards.

Each headline issue is represented in a table formatted to present content information. Below is an example that conveys the issue of social exclusion (see Table 6.3).

The information card starts with the headline issue and a brief description in the top two rows. In the bottom two rows we see links to other headline cards in two boxes: one relating to other headline social concerns, the other to headline personal concerns. In the third row we have bulleted individual issues. These are briefly described, so for example an important contributory aspect to social exclusion is geographical isolation, most commonly felt by those who live in rural areas. This geographical distance is closely related to local transport provision. This is represented in the 'related social concerns' row of the table because there it is another headline issue. In turn geographical isolation and transport provision relate directly to the personal concern of personal mobility, seen in the 'related personal concerns' row. Again because this has wider implications and is complex in and of itself, it too is a headline issue, this time under the category of personal concerns. Other detailed elements include the person being homebound, joined up services and early intervention. As can be seen the social exclusion card is related to a number of other headline issues including housing provision, wealth and poverty, social contact, fear of crime, social participation, social care provision.

Table 6.3. The information card for social exclusion

Headline issue	**SOCIAL EXCLUSION**
Brief description	The process whereby certain groups are pushed to the margins of society and prevented from participating
Pages expanding on this issue (click for more)	• Geographical/rural isolation • Homebound individuals • Early intervention: before a crisis occurs • Joined up service provision in the social services • Identifying and helping the 'most excluded'
References	Social Exclusion Unit 'Excluded Older People' June 2005 Evans G (2005) Accessibility and user needs in transport design. In: International Conference on Inclusive Design, Royal College of Art, London, UK
Related Social concerns (click)	Transport provision; Housing provision; Wealth and poverty;
Related Personal concerns (click)	Personal mobility; Social contact; Fear of crime; Social participation; Social care; Personal care;

The objective of Table 6.3 then is to give an overview of the variety of issues facing and contributing to social exclusion in a brief and accessible format. For each of the elements in the 'Detail' row that are not linked to other headline issues, there is a information card, which contains relevant information, quotations and statistics, examples, and the like. To give a flavour of the content we have included below an abbreviated version of the card relating to the detailed element of 'early intervention' (see Table 6.4).

The way we envisage a designer using the resource is to start from the list of headline issues and then access one information card and then link either sideways to either other social or personal headline information cards or downwards to the detailed information card.

Table 6.4. A table showing an information card

Detailed concern	**EARLY INTERVENTION**
Description and information: The government maintains that intervening early through low-level preventative methods can lead to a better quality of life for older people, who can live in their homes for longer. Lack of early prevention is one of three key issues identified in the recent government report entitled 'Excluded Older People' (2005). Early intervention involves efforts to offset or avoid later problems by recognising the 'symptoms' of social exclusion, such as retreat into own home after death of spouse. "When thinking about older people there is a tendency (quite logically) to concentrate on people of a certain age of over, typically 65. However many of the problems that lead to social exclusion have their roots in an earlier stage of life and so the report examines issues felt by those between 50 and 65 that may result in social exclusion later in life" (Ibid). There is a financial incentive as well; 'Much of the social care that is available is focused on expensive nursing care rather than low level early interventions which would make it easier for people to live at home' (Ibid. p.15). The alternative is to provide for 'low level interventions': "Intervening early is important, and investment in low level prevention can reduce costlier interventions later." (Ibid. p.6). Diagram adapted from the Joseph Rowntree Foundation: **Physical and practical** **Home:** Heating/insulation, Home safety/security, Cleaning, Shopping, Gardening, Equipment, Adaptations, Home Improvement Agencies, Community Alarms, Use of technology, Handyperson/repairs, Lifetime housing, **Environment:** Transport, Personal safety, Street lighting, Built environment (pavements, dropped kerbs, disabled access), Traffic management, Community centres, Advice centres and one stop shops, Accessible shops with affordable products. **Personal and Social** **Home:** Befriending, Bathing, Meals service, Hairdressing, Carers support, Range of personal care including nursing, Intensive home support, Resettlement into sheltered housing, Floating support, Rapid response, Rehabilitation, Advocacy. **Environment:** Leisure, Primary Health care, Chiropody, Lifelong learning, Libraries, Employment, Volunteering, Day care, Luncheon clubs, Rehabilitation, Community development, Healthy living schemes, Peer support.	
Possible responses: In addition to provision of low level services above: better monitoring of people's needs at an earlier stage; systems interventions for the younger aged that can develop in response to changing needs.	

The current table and hypertext design is applicable to a variety of resources. One idea is to present the material online as a form of "wiki" so that new examples can be added by different people and additional notes added as the material is applied.

As can be seen the 'headline' issue of social exclusion is highly complex. Not only is social exclusion related to issues such as mobility, public transport provision and geographical isolation, but these factors are inter-related, such that geographical isolation emphasises the need for public transport provision to counter immobility. One key insight is that these issues have multiple factors themselves and therefore we are encouraged to think about layered and relational solutions. One way to formulate layered and relational solutions is to think about services that involve multiple actors utilizing a variety of technologies.

6.5 Technological Responses to Social Exclusion

This section illustrates how social and psychological issues can motivate new design. The example emerged from user-centred research at the University of York. An ethnography of older people and care services identified a number of high level issues facing socially excluded older individuals, including a lack of mobility and the inability to shop for themselves. Shopping of course is a social activity and these individuals were not only physically isolated, but socially isolated too, with little human contact. It was realised that any response would necessarily be layered and so a service was invented that combined both befriending and shopping. The response, the Net Neighbours Scheme enables older people in the York region to effectively shop on-line without direct access to a computer. The scheme uses volunteers to act as intermediaries to on-line shopping at the main supermarkets based in York. The volunteer contacts the client and takes a shopping order over the phone, and then at their own computer inputs the details and places the order. Also the volunteer spends time chatting to the client. Age Concern York (ACY) administer the service, and bring together individual volunteers and individual clients as part of their broader professional role. They recruit the clients and volunteers to the service and provide training and guidance where necessary. The supermarket makes up the order and a member of delivery staff delivers the goods. The client sends a cheque or cash to ACY, who then reimburse the volunteer. (Blythe *et al.*, 2004; Baxter *et al.*, 2005).

The system has a number of advantages: (1) it targets the concerns of the stakeholders involved. These include the older client, concerned about social isolation and lack of social contact, the volunteers who wishes to participate socially, the care professional wishing to provide additional services, and the supermarket's wish to reach a new customer base. (2) vitally, it targets and brings together the capacites of the various stakeholders; the capacity of the client to use the telephone, the computer skills of the volunteer, and the mobility of the delivery service. (3) and finally, it is a distributed socio-technical system that is complex, yet provides for real needs in a layered and relational way.

The service is presented below as a rich picture, a methodology taken from an approach within HCI called soft systems methodology (SSM) originally developed by Checkland (1981) and developed here by Monk (1998). The purpose of a rich picture is to detail the concerns of those stakeholders involved, and one way that it can be used is as a means to brainstorm system design.

We have developed the method to include stakeholders' broad social and psychological concerns as well as their concerns about the system itself (shown in italics). Further, each set of stakeholders is detailed in terms of their relevant capacities, whether they be related to general life skills or to technology. In this way it is possible to see how the concerns of one set of stakeholders might be addressed by the capacties of another. Through sensitive system design we match the various technological elements of the system to the people, rather than developing a new system with completely new technology elements. In this way we do what might be called *capacity matching*.

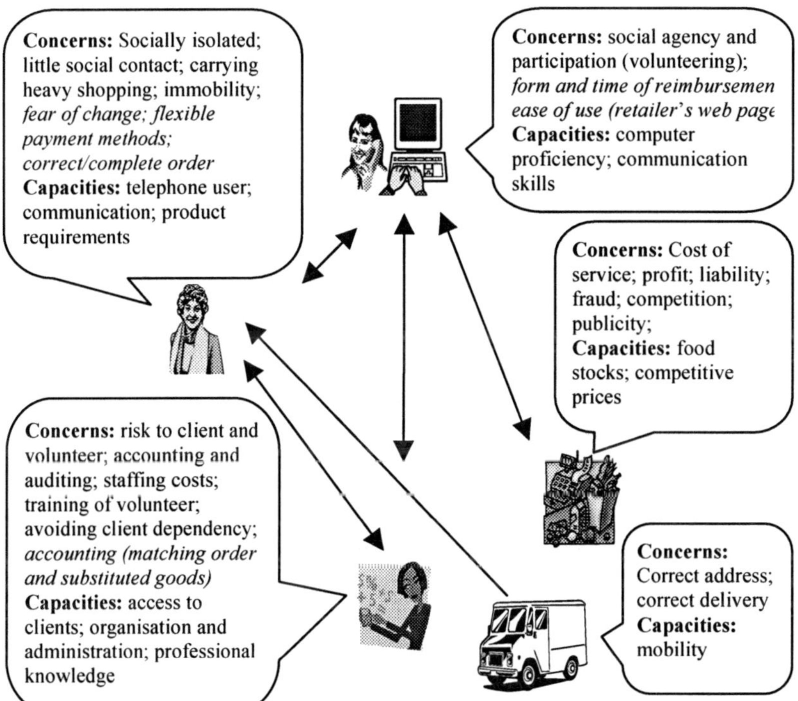

Figure 6.1. A rich picture showing the stakeholders of the Net Neighbours Service and stakeholder concerns and capacities

An example of capacity matching can be seen in a comparison of the client's concerns and the capacities of the supermarket's delivery service. The first has limited mobility, the second is by its nature mobile. Similarly the volunteers concern to participate is matched with the client's needs for release from social isolation through interpersonal contact. Perhaps most interesting is the technological capacity matching seen in the relationships. The capacity of the client to use the telephone and the capactity of the volunteer to use the computer combine and then integrate with the supermarket's capactity to provide and maintain retail website that links directly to their products. ACY's administrative capacities and continued work with the client group (arguably an administrative technology) bring all these features together and ensure their continued viability.

We can see how the Net Neighbours Scheme meets the criteria of a layered and relational solution to complex high level issues. We could imagine other volunteer based internet services, such as the provision of travel information. Also it is built upon current technology, the telephone and retail web sites, but as new technologies become available, such as voice over IP we could imagine services such as a volunteer based chat service for older people; provided currently by specialised charities (see Reed, 2003) in which the telephone and internet services combine. Once we start to engage with wider social and psychological issues and have tools to reason about system design, we can address these broad concerns and issues.

6.6 Conclusions

We started this paper by asking about the definition of inclusive design and suggested an alternative formulation of design for inclusion. By prioritizing the social and personal concerns of older people, and presenting this information in a formalised template, we aim to provide a resource for understanding the complex layered and relational character of such problems. Using the net neighbours scheme as an example of a distributed socio-technical system that targets the concerns and capacities of different stakeholders, we gave an example of how such complex issues might be addressed through a user-centred mentality, and how future service based interventions may be developed.

Inclusive Design should do more than extend the reach of mainstream technology and the popularity of assistive devices, it should fulfill its political underpinnings and orient to the broader needs of the excluded of society. We have suggested the notion of *design for inclusion* as an alternative formulation of inclusive design, but of course we are not suggesting that the first replace the second.

A consequence of thinking about design for inclusion is that we start to think about high level issues such as social exclusion and formulate in reply high level responses. This removes the burden of having to make every device inclusive, and releases us from debates about specificality and universality. Instead our responses can be formulated above the single or even multiple device level and incorporate people as well as technologies. In a sense such high level approaches provide a solution for the integration of the specific and the universal through a form of User Centred Design, that understands individuals in a matrix of relationships whose consequences and outcomes are inclusive. In return a wealth of responses open up, including commercial and social services that combine and integrate technology and practice.

6.7 References

Balaram S (2001) Universal design and the majority world. In: Preiser WFE, Ostroff E (eds.) Universal design handbook. McGraw-Hill, New York, UK

Baxter GB, Arief B, Smith S, Monk A (2005) Structuring dependable on-line services: a case study using internet grocery shopping. In: Proceedings of the 5th Annual DIRC Research Conference, Lancaster, UK

Blythe M, Monk A, Baxter G, Jarred J (2004) Making a net neighbours service. Available at: http://www-users.york.ac.uk/~am1/Making.PDF

Checkland P (1981) Systems thinking, systems practice. John Wiley, Chichester, UK

D'Souza N (2004) Is universal design a critical theory? In: Proceedings of CWUAAT'04, Cambridge, UK

Evans G (2005) Accessibility and user needs in transport design. In: Proceedings of INCLUDE 2005, Royal College of Art, London, UK

Hawthorn D (2003) How universal is good design for older users. In: Proceedings of CUU'03, Vancouver, Canada

Hirsch T, Forlizzi J, Hyder E, Goetz J, Stroback J *et al.* (2000) The ELDer project: social, emotional, and environmental factors in the design of eldercare technologies. In: Proceedings of CUU'00, Arlington, USA

Keates S, Clarkson J, Langdon P, Robinson P (eds.) (2004) Designing a more inclusive world. Springer, London, UK

Monk A (1998) Lightweight techniques to encourage innovative user interface design. In: Wood L (ed.) User interface design: bridging the gap from user requirements to design. CRC Press, Boca Raton, USA

Newell AF (2003) Inclusive design or assistive technology. In: Clarkson PJ *et al.* (eds.) Inclusive design: design for the whole population. Springer, London, UK

Newell AF, Gregor P (2000) User sensitive inclusive design – in search of a new paradigm. In: Proceedings of CUU'00, Arlington, USA

Newell AF, Monk A (2006) Involving older people in the design of IT systems. In: Clarkson PJ *et al.* Design for inclusivity. Gower (in press)

Reed DJ (2003) Fun on the phone. The situated experience of recreational telephone conferences. In: Blythe M *et al.* (eds.) From usability to enjoyment. Kluwer, London, UK

Chapter 7

Designers' Use of the Artefact in Human-centred Design

P.M. Chamberlain and S.J. Bowen

7.1 Introduction

This paper highlights how artefacts can be used as an effective tool to understand users and encourage dialogue. The paper will reflect on how the role of the designer is evolving, some limitations of user-centred design and how a more holistic 'human-centred' design approach may be more productive. The nature and applications of artefacts in understanding users will be considered. Finally three case studies will illustrate how artefacts have been used to enable human-centred design.

The authors work within the Art and Design Research Centre at Sheffield Hallam University (SHU). South Yorkshire has a world-wide tradition in the heavy industries of steel and coal but has witnessed its workforce in these industries decline by over 70% since the late eighties – there are now no deep mines in the region. The Art and Design Research Centre has played a significant role via collaborations with local industry to take help regenerate, redefine and reinforce industry within the region. The authors are design researchers who through fundamental and then applied research programmes are making a considerable contribution to industrial product development. Previous projects such as the use of waste glass (Roddis and Chamberlain, 1999) and the following case studies demonstrate how the design researchers have 'joined forces', establishing collaborative alliances between designers, clients/manufacturers, users, and 'other stakeholders', and provide examples of the designer as the 'mobiliser' of new solutions. Key to this approach is the multi-disciplinary nature of the research undertaken. Prof. Rachel Cooper, Editorial Chair of the internationally refereed Design Journal, recently referred to a paper based on a case study of their work (Chamberlain and Roddis, 2003). She says, "If we are to consider the future of design methodology, this is a good example of the trend of design leading research in collaboration with social and scientific disciplines".

7.2 The Role of the Designer

Designing is not an insular activity: designers need to engage with users and specialists from other disciplines. Design, unlike many disciplines, is not governed or restricted by context. However, some perceptions about the role of the designer in new product development need re-evaluating. The relationships between designers, users and other stakeholders are evolving.

7.2.1 Beyond Styling

There is increasing literature on new product development (NPD) processes which aims to provide models of practice and identify factors that account for success. A shortcoming of most of this literature is that it assumes design to be a functional resource directed by management strategically to enhance the NPD process. Much of this literature is produced to educate business managers, so it is hardly surprising that it conceptualises NPD as a corporate-driven process which employs the services of design.

Design is often seen as a resource to embellish products towards the end of the research and development process. Once the science has been established and the engineering proven, designers are brought in to add visual value to a product. A traditional view of the industrial design profession is that it tends to be preoccupied with *visual* appearance, at the expense of other factors. In the USA, the first industrial designers were known as 'stylists' since their chief concern was the cosmetic appearance of products (Margolin, 1997; Rothstein, 2000).

However, Jevnaker (1998) does provide different models of 'design alliances', one of which – entrepreneurial mobilisation – considers the role of the designer as a "dialectical, knowledge-intensive, source of innovation" who can take on an entrepreneurial role in the process. Despite high profile examples of design as 'entrepreneurial mobilisation', such as Sir Terence Conran or James Dyson, there are few analytical case studies available.

7.2.2 User-centred Design

'User-centred' design methods have been widely discussed within product design discourse, and also in the disciplines of human computer interaction (HCI), human factors engineering and ergonomics. McDonagh-Philp (1998) suggests the following definition of user-centred design:

> *"User-centred design is a design methodology that utilises the target product users as a designing resource to increase the understanding of the design practitioner."*

Many business models will assume an understanding can be established through marketing techniques and questionnaires. However there has to be a clear understanding of users' needs and wants. Henry Ford is supposed to have said: "If I had asked people what they wanted, they would have said faster horses".

Questionnaires can confirm past prejudices and breed mediocrity and dullness. Would the Wright brothers have invented the aeroplane on basis of a questionnaire, or Edison the light bulb?

If the aim is to improve the usability of products, it is essential that designers acquire knowledge of product use that is derived from first hand experience. In some cases, such as when designing familiar consumer products, designers can draw on their own 'real-life' experience of using these products. It is therefore necessary for designers to build close collaborative relationships with product users and, where possible, to take part in user activities themselves:

> *"I have washed clothes, cooked, driven a tractor, run a Diesel locomotive, spread manure, vacuumed rugs, and ridden in an armoured tank. I have operated a sewing machine, a telephone switchboard, a corn picker, a lift truck, a turret lathe, and a linotype machine. [..] We ride in submarines and jet planes. All this in the name of research."*
>
> (Dreyfuss, 1955)

However, this approach becomes difficult when designing products outside the designers' or users' experience; products with unfamiliar contexts, applications or enabling technologies, for users with different capabilities and impairments or where users' safety may be at risk.

7.2.3 Human-centred Design

In certain situations it is difficult to define who the 'user' is. For example who are the users of assistive technology? The patient; the carer; the patient's family; the therapist; the teacher; the local community; the healthcare trust?

Human-centred design is a broader concept; a holistic approach that explores the relationships between the designer, the various end-users, and the other 'stakeholders' within the system of production and consumption. This may include those who manufacture, transport, sell, carry out maintenance, or dispose of the product or system at the end of its useful working life. The role of the designer becomes that of 'advocate' within a system of production and consumption that is socially and ethically responsible (Papanek, 1971).

A challenge to this approach is establishing communication methods that provide a clear understanding between the potentially diverse users and stakeholders involved. This entails enabling the communication of information and ideas, sometimes unusual or challenging, between specialisms and between specialists and non-specialists via a common language. A designer must understand the technical, commercial and personal 'jargon' of the users and stakeholders to both develop the questions and then appreciate and understand what the answers mean.

7.3 The Role of the Artefact

The Oxford English Dictionary (2002) defines an artefact as "an object made by a human being" (2002). The variety of manufacturable 'objects' means that artefacts are not restricted to physical but may also take virtual forms – as electronic media and interactive experiences. Artefacts reflect the knowledge, intent and ideas of their maker(s). Thus artefacts can be effective vehicles for communication: to make statements, encapsulate ideas and illustrate knowledge.

Dunne (1999) suggests "conceptual design objects" as a way of expressing unusual ideas and challenging technology's roles and applications. The objects are not intended as practical prototypes but rather "encourage complex and meaningful reflection" (1999) of the hypotheses they represent. Gaver and Martin (2000) apply such artefacts as a way of "mapping the design space", exploring the territory where future solutions could be positioned.

Gaver *et al.* (1999) use artefacts as "Cultural Probes" to gather information. Users are presented with a miscellany of artefacts with which to record their views and experiences. The design and selection of these probes pose deliberately ambiguous questions prompting rich subjective interaction and identification of needs.

Rust (2004) discusses the concept of 'tacit knowledge' – knowledge that is fundamentally embedded in action and may not be readily explained by explicit reasoning, for example a craftsperson's 'feel' for shaping wood. Interaction with artefacts provides an environment in which users' tacit knowledge can be revealed. Rust suggests that creating artefacts "can give us access to tacit knowledge, and can stimulate people to employ their tacit knowledge to form new ideas".

Design provides ways of thinking and skills that can deliver artefacts as tools for creating new scenarios of the world we live in. These scenarios can simulate unfamiliar experiences and allow users to make imaginative extensions into unfamiliar areas. Thus designers can create new 'contexts' for others to experience and explore as part of human-centred design.

7.4 Case Studies

7.4.1 Multi-sensory Design: Tac-tile Sounds System™

This project was concerned with the design and development of sensory equipment for people with profound sensory disability and with its therapeutic, educational and recreational benefits. It was conducted through the Art and Design Research Centre's collaborative initiatives with clinicians, musicians, technologists and latterly Rompa – one of the leading suppliers of products and equipment for special needs teaching and sensory environments. Design-led research projects resulted in product outcomes that were subsequently adopted by Rompa and have since achieved major design awards (Design Council, 2000). The relationship with the company has led to the establishment of a sensory research centre within the University.

Early stages of research and development involved a process of collaboration and communication between the design team directed by Paul Chamberlain, a team of clinical and educational specialists and the end-users, who in the main were deaf children and, in some cases, deaf-blind. In short, the problem was that the design team was faced with the challenges of understanding highly specialised fields of clinical and educational practice, and the end-users literally could not hear what the designers and the clinicians were trying to achieve. Somehow the designers had to develop methods of communication that went beyond words. It was quite literally through 'feelings and vibrations' provided by artefacts that the research team gained the knowledge necessary to develop the product. The artefacts became the vehicle for communication between the designers, end-users and specialists.

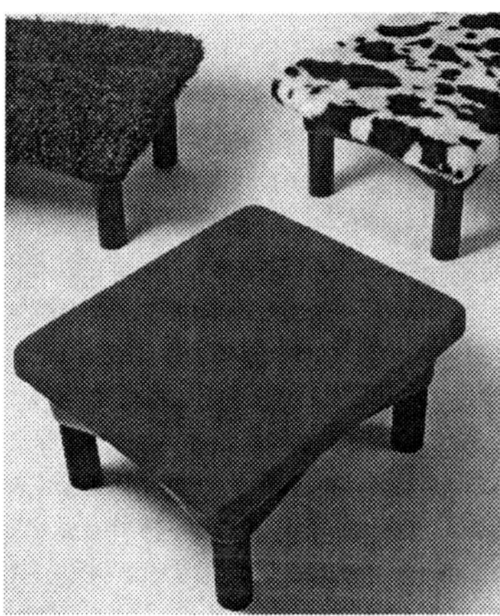

Figure 7.1. *Tac-tile sounds system*™

An early development from this research was a versatile vibro-acoustic modular system that tries to convey the emotions of music and meaningful sounds to people who cannot hear in the usual way. The product, now manufactured and marketed as the *tac-tile sounds system*™, (Rompa) is a system that delivers sounds to a series of resonating surfaces where they are converted into mechanical vibrations which can be felt by people who cannot hear sounds in the usual way. The system has a wide range of uses in clinical, rehabilitation, educational and domestic settings.

It is interesting to note that 'key partners' in the sensory research were initially clinicians, Derbyshire Health Authority's Ashgreen Centre, a residential and special day care centre and Russ Palmer, a Music therapist who himself is deaf/blind. These key partners provided access to other important specialists and users to input useful information to the project. The Design team liaised with technical specialists to inform the project and the Music Department at the University of Sheffield to compose 'low frequency' music for the system. The manufacturers, Rompa, were a 'sub partner' who only engaged in the research at the latter stages of realisation when the work had been trialled and tested.

As our research has progressed Rompa have become a 'key partner' and have now formally 'joined forces' with the Art and Design Research Centre at Sheffield

Hallam University. The *Everysense* system multi-sensory environment (Rompa) is a product of this ongoing research collaboration.

7.4.2 Haptic Design: Medical Connectors

Paul Chamberlain is currently leading a research project funded by the Department of Health, with B.Braun Medical, a major international medical device company, to minimise medical misconnection errors through the design of a non interchangeable medical connector system. The project has produced generalizable knowledge about haptic affordances and a methodology for evaluating them, which may inform the design of other safety critical control systems.

The increasing complexity of medical interventions and the associated medical devices means that users are required to connect a multiplicity of external tubes to various types of diagnostic and therapeutic devices. A typical patient in a coronary care unit may have as many as 40 connectors. It is not surprising then that errors arise. Recent incidents that have led to patient fatalities where drugs were administered intrathecally (via the spine) that should have been delivered intravenously (into the vein) have raised concern about the application of a single connector design to a number of incompatible applications. Our research brings together a multidisciplinary team to design and test a new system of medical connectors. There is now significant pressure for research and development into a system of medical connectors that will distinguish between the different routes of delivery, so that misconnections of this kind become physically impossible. The design of a non-interchangeable connector system will eliminate the possibility of misconnection, which has the potential for catastrophic results. Currently more people die through medical errors than in motor related accidents. An easily identifiable system should eliminate the common practice of customised labelling and reduce the time for clinical checking procedures. Clinical practice will benefit in terms of a safer, time saving system which should contribute to a less stressful working environment. The project will lead to a new range of innovative devices and could provide valuable new knowledge that will inform their future product development

The research brings together expertise in general and regional anaesthesia, critical care medicine (Bradford Royal Infirmary), psychology and human factors (University of Leeds) and industrial design (Sheffield Hallam University) to develop an engineered design solution supported by a *novel* means of enhancing the discriminability of a new system of connectors through visual and tactile (haptic) cues. B.Braun Medical, a major international manufacturer and supplier to the health industry, provides technical expertise and will support the route to market.

A key research challenge was to devise methods to evaluate visual and haptic discriminations and affordances. The concept of an affordance was coined by the perceptual psychologist James J. Gibson (1979) in his seminal book *The ecological approach to visual perception.* According to Norman (1988) an affordance is the design aspect of an object which suggest how the object should be used; a visual clue to its function and use. How could the connectors' shape and texture aid identification and afford their use and method of connection? A varied set of connectors was designed and presented to users who were given timed tasks to identify their affordances (push or twist). CAD simulations were used to test visual affordances and physical prototypes were used to test and compare haptic affordances. These artefacts therefore simulated new user experiences for study. The research team realised "conducting user-based research in the setting of an intensive care ward was going to be an ethical and practical minefield" (Walters *et al.*, 2003): using simulated experiences allowed such problems to be avoided.

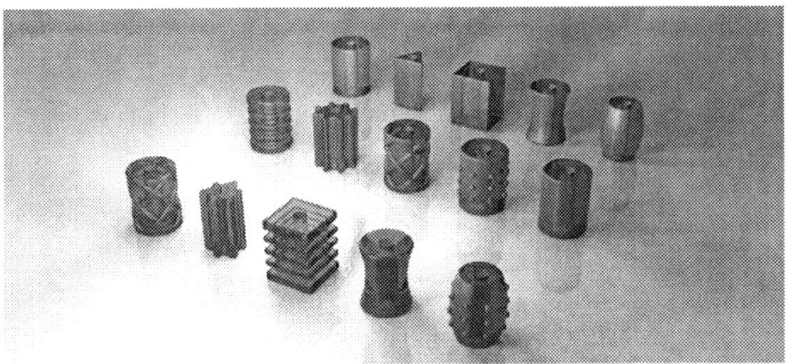

Figure 7.2. CAD rendering of prototype medical connectors using shape and texture as a means of discrimination

7.4.3 Ideation: Digital Photograph Collections

Simon Bowen's MA work investigated methods for involving users in the identification of new product opportunities for new technologies; how to make users key participants in the ideation process. The project produced a hypothetical methodology that he is investigating further via a PhD.

User groups representing older people and families with young children were chosen to explore the specific context of the roles and management of digital family photograph collections. The increasing number of digital photographs taken is creating an information management problem:

> *"Having thousands of photos on a hard disk or DVD-ROM is the equivalent of throwing [..] images into the air and letting them flutter to the ground."*
>
> (Weinberger, 2004)

Rapidly developing digital technologies are becoming increasingly pervasive and offer numerous possibilities to enhance our lives. The social role technology occupies in our lives is changing. So how can new applications for these technologies be determined that accurately reflect users' wants and needs?

Early sessions using questionnaires, interviews and low-fidelity prototyping (after Ehn and Kyng, 1991) produced limited results. Users had difficulty articulating their needs or exploring new contexts in an unfamiliar territory – the application of new technologies, such as wireless networking and electronic ink displays, to photograph collections. Being biased by familiar experience users generally asked for 'faster horses'.

A more productive approach was to use a set of conceptual designs (after Dunne, 1999) in workshops with users. The artefacts were created to embody various (occasionally provocative) ideas, values and needs, and their presentation allowed the imaginative extension of users' experiences that could then be explored. Users' interaction with the artefacts provided rich, qualitative data – what was liked or disliked, what was appropriate or inappropriate. The artefacts proposed a position in the 'design space' of potential new products. This created a dialogue with users that intimated where the location of actual new products might be.

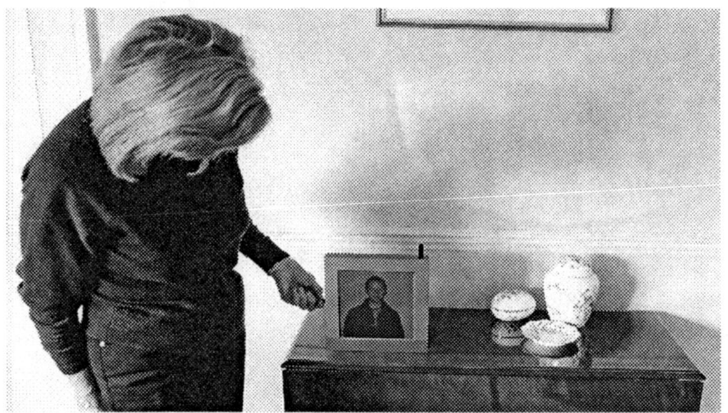

Figure 7.3. *Forget Me Not Frame* conceptual design

For example the *Forget Me Not Frame* concept displays a photograph that fades over time with a lever that can restore it. Users' strong dislike of this feature highlighted the need to feel in control of such emotive subject matter; users did not want the presence of personal photographs to be automated.

The project yielded several 'way marker' concepts indicating directions for further product development in the specific context. A more general methodology for using artefacts in the ideation process of user-centred product development also began to emerge. Simon is now developing this methodology via AHRC-funded doctoral research.

7.5 Conclusions

The role of designer has evolved considerably from adding 'styling' to products towards the end of their development. Designers can be the mobilisers of new solutions, advocates within multi-disciplinary teams and involved throughout the research and development process.

Traditional immersive user research techniques have limitations. It is difficult to understand users' needs and wants in scenarios that are outside their experience.

Designers can use artefacts to create new contexts for study – enabling users to explore unfamiliar territory.

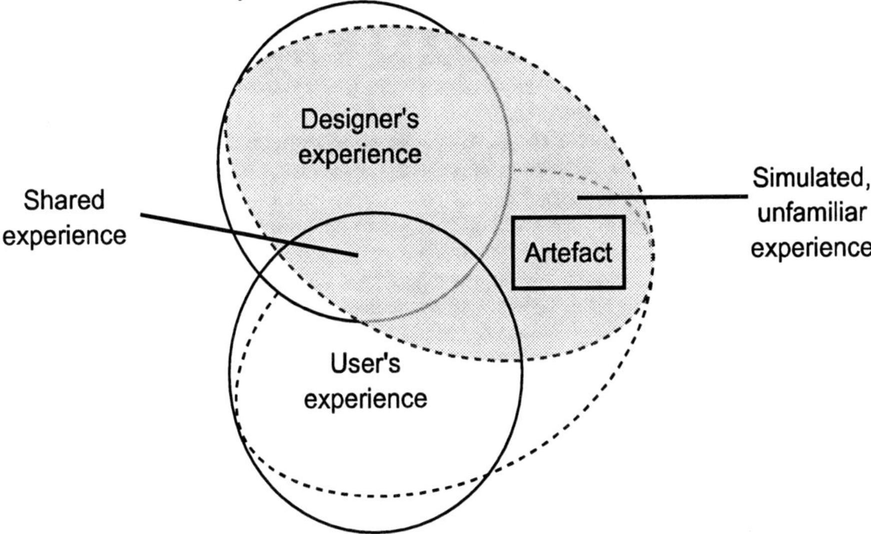

Figure 7.4. The artefact used to extend the designer's and user's experiences

The question of who is 'the user' covers an increasing number of roles. Human-centred design offers a more holistic approach considering all the diverse types of users and stakeholders of a product. Artefacts can be used as vehicles for communication in such situations where traditional methods may be inadequate.

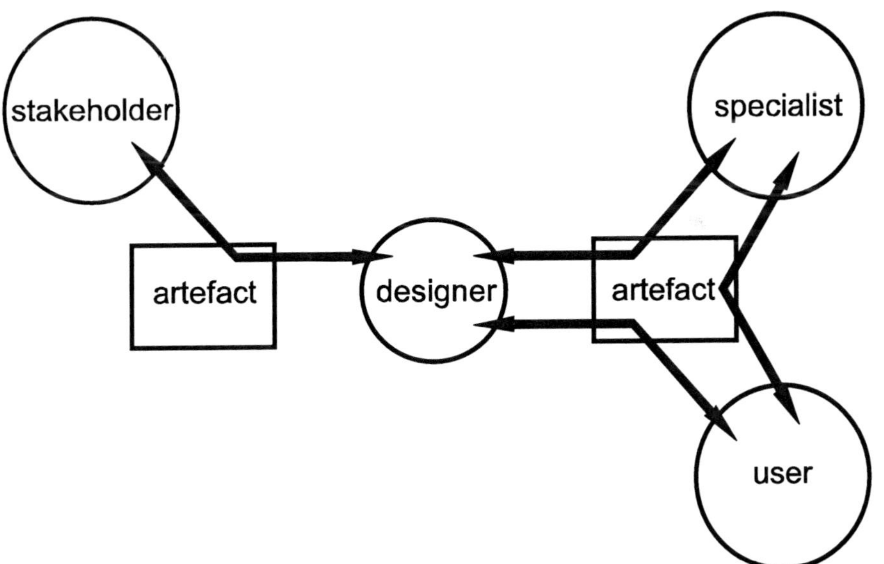

Figure 7.5. The artefact as a vehicle for communication in multi-disciplinary teams

7.6 References

Chamberlain P, Roddis J (2003) Making sense: a case study in collaborative design-led new product development for the sensorial impaired. The Design Journal 6(1): 40–51

Design Council (2000) Millennium products – tac-tile sounds system and Q chair. Available at: http://tinyurl.com/9bose

Dreyfuss H (1955) Designing for people. Grossman Publishers, New York, USA

Dunne A (1999) Hertzian tales – electronic products, aesthetic experience and critical design. Royal College of Art, UK

Ehn P, Kyng M (1991) Cardboard computers: mocking-it-up or hands-on the future. In: Greenbaum J, Kyng M (eds.) Design at work: cooperative design of computer systems. Lawrence Erlbaum Associates, New Jersey, USA

Gaver B, Dunne A, Pacenti E (1999) Cultural probes. Interactions 6(1): 21–29

Gaver B, Martin H (2000) Exploring information appliances through conceptual design proposals. In: Proceedings of CHI 2000, ACM Press

Gibson JJ (1979) The ecological approach to visual perception. Lawrence Erlbaum Associates, New Jersey, USA

Jevnaker B (1998) Absorbing or creating design ability: HAG, HAMAX and TOMRA. In: Bruce B, Jevnaker M (eds.) Managing design alliances. John Wiley, Chicester, UK

Margolin V (1997) Getting to know the user. Design Studies 18(3): 227–236

McDonagh-Philp D (1998) Gender and design: towards an appropriate research methodology. In: Proceedings of the 5th National Conference on Product Design Education, Glamorgan University, Wales, UK

Norman DA (1988) The design of everyday things. Doubleday, New York, USA

Oxford University Dictionary (2002) Concise Oxford English Dictionary. Oxford University Press

Papanek V (1971) Design for the real world – human ecology and social change. Thames and Hudson, London, UK

Roddis J, Chamberlain P (1999) Furniture design and the environment, innovation and legislation. A case study of a design-led research programme investigating the use of waste glass in open-loop solutions. In: Proceedings of the International Furniture Congress, Istanbul Technical University, Turkey

Rompa. Available at: http://www.rompa.com/cgi-bin/Rompa.storefront

Rothstein P (2000) Ethnographic research: teaching a young profession old tricks. Innovation (Winter): 33–38

Rust C (2004) Design enquiry: tacit knowledge and invention. Science Design Issues 20(4): 76–85

Walters P, Chamberlain P, Press M (2003) In touch: an investigation of the benefits of tactile cues in safety-critical product applications. In: Proceedings of the 5th European Academy of Design Conference, Barcelona University, Spain

Weinberger D (2004) Point. Shoot. Kiss it good-bye. Wired 12(10): 148–152

Part II

Enabling Computer Access and the Development of New Technologies

Chapter 8

Introducing COGAIN – Communication by Gaze Interaction

R. Bates, M. Donegan, H.O. Istance, J.P. Hansen and K.-J. Räihä

8.1 Introducing COGAIN

Communication by Gaze Interaction (COGAIN) is a European research Network of Excellence (NoE), which is aimed specifically at enabling rapid and natural communication and control via eye gaze for users with high-level motor disabilities. The aim of this presentation is to introduce the work of COGAIN and to freely offer the services and expertise of COGAIN to users, workers in the field, and researchers so that we may work together to enable greater communication by eye gaze for high-level motor disabled users.

COGAIN consists of researchers and industries from 20 universities, institutions and industries from across Europe that have come together in a 3 million Euro 5 year project to develop new ways of enabling communication, environmental control, and personal mobility all based solely on using eye gaze. The project focuses on improving the quality of life for those whose life is impaired by motor-control disorders, such as Amyotrophic Lateral Sclerosis (ALS) or Cerebral Palsy (CP), by developing gaze driven assistive technologies that will empower users to communicate by using the capabilities they have, and by offering compensation for capabilities that are deteriorating, all at a completely new level of convenience and speed via gaze-based communication.

COGAIN has four main aims – to form outreach groups and networks to work with disabled users, workers in the field and rehabilitation centres to assess and identify their communication and control needs and abilities, to use these findings to develop new methods and systems for communication and control by eye gaze, to produce new hardware and software eye driven systems that are for the first time both low-cost and freely available, and finally to call for users and researchers interested in eye gaze communication to work with COGAIN and exploit our resources and outcomes in a combined effort toward greater and more enabling technologies for motor disabled users.

8.2 The Motivation for COGAIN

The ability to express oneself quickly and efficiently in a precise language is fundamental to quality of life; however some people with high-level motor disabilities such as ALS or locked-in syndrome are not able to carry out such interpersonal communication fluently. For example, due to a lack of control over movement many motor disabled users may find efficient communication extremely difficult and frustrating, with some users almost unable to communicate in conventional ways due to their disabilities. Similarly, user requirements of technology and communication such as access to the information society through the Internet may be severely limited or be impractical by an inability to use the normal controls of a computer. These problems are compounded by limitations in the range of currently available eye-enabled applications, resulting in a greatly reduced uptake of eye gaze by disabled users (Jordansen *et al.,* 2005), (Figure 8.1). Addressing these profound communication needs of users with high-level disabilities is the motivation behind the COGAIN network.

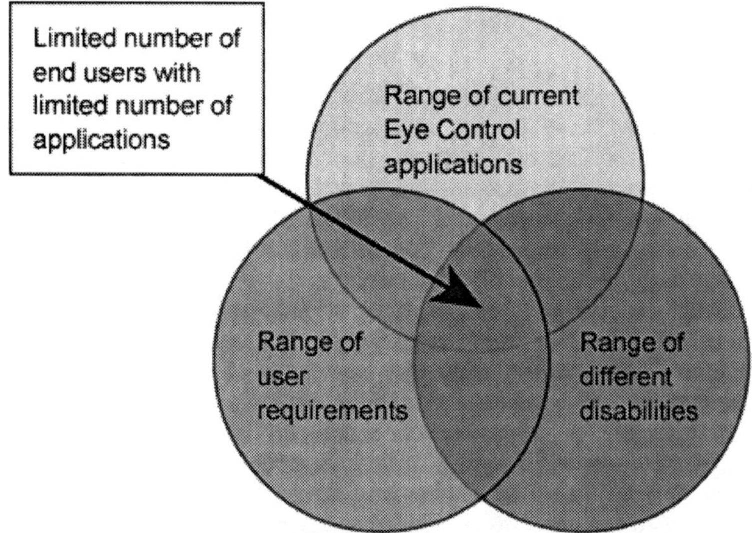

Figure 8.1. Current restrictions of eye gaze communication

8.3 The Benefits of Gaze Communication

The benefits of eye gaze communication can be illustrated by case study, as the information acquired from users provides a valuable insight into the impact of eye control technology on quality of life, and valuable direction for eye gaze control research both within COGAIN, and across a wider field of research areas.

8.3.1 Birger

Birger suffers from ALS and now, due to progressing motor paralysis, can only communicate with a few trained professional carers via tiny eye brow movements, producing words and commands slowly by spelling and intuition (Figure 8.2, left). However, by using the latest eye gaze communication software from COGAIN Birger can now communicate effectively via eye gaze using an on-screen keyboard. It is a clear demonstration of the enabling power of eye gaze – with this system he can type text and email freely (Figure 8.2, right) and surf the internet all without any help – opportunities that were impossible before his eye gaze communication system was developed. An informative video illustrating user needs, the communication difficulties experienced by high-level motor disabled users, and the benefits of gaze based communication in empowering communication and quality of life is shown accompanying this presentation ('Communicating by the Eyes' is available via www.cogain.org)

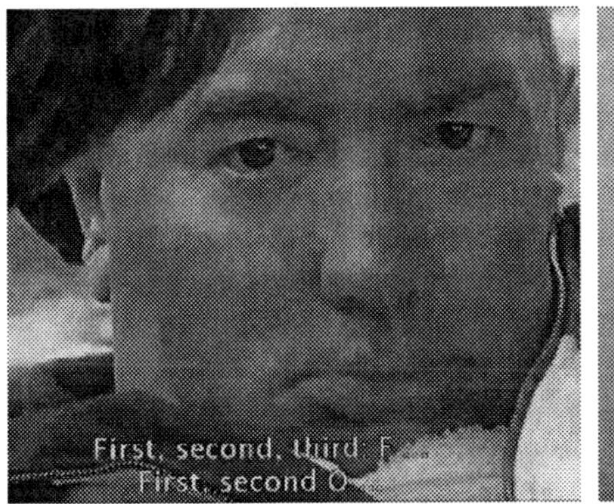

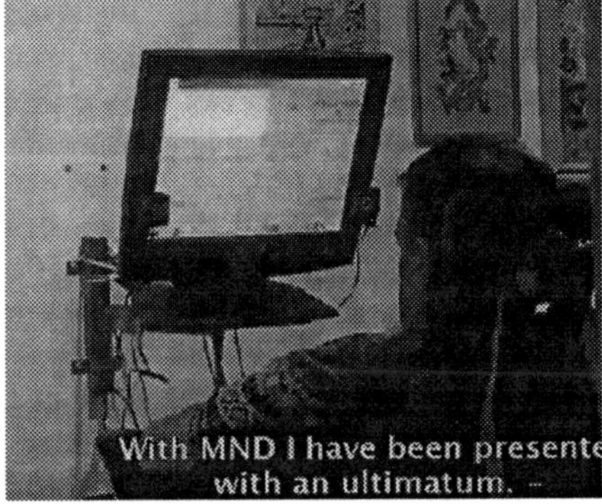

Figure 8.2. Birger communicating by eyebrow movement, and typing by eye gaze alone

8.3.2 Keith

Keith has ALS and is completely paralysed, being only able to move his eyes. He can no longer move his head at all, and he cannot blink, making communication extremely difficult. He now uses an eye tracking system for communication extensively, often up to 12 hours daily.

Keith now regards eye-control of his computer as essential to his quality of life: "I would have no desire to live without this eye-gaze system", and uses it for a range of activities, such as social communication, writing, emailing and access to the Internet. Eye-writing using an on-screen gaze driven keyboard is his "only way of communicating". It enables him to "still be a part of other people's lives. Plus, I can still give advice and help others". Through emailing, he keeps in daily contact with people: "It gives me an outlet to feel like I can still make a difference on somebody's life". The Internet is his "only way of keeping up with what's going on in the outside world". Eye-writing is quicker for him than when he was able to use his fingers to type: “I am faster with my eyes than I ever was when my fingers used to work”.

Keith has asked COGAIN researchers if it would be possible for him to control his wheelchair using his eyes, as it would provide him with “freedom from always having to ask others for help”. He would also like to be able to use eye-gaze to take control over his environment “so I could be more independent…to change TV channels, turn lights on and answer the phone”. From input by Keith and others, both personal mobility and personal environmental control are now solutions that are being addressed by COGAIN researchers.

8.3.3 Claire

Claire has athetoid cerebral palsy, which means it is very difficult for her to control her movements. She is very bright, literate and well motivated. She uses a special joystick to access the computer. Using the joystick and a range of specialised on-screen grids she is able to use the joystick effectively and accurately to control the computer. Nonetheless, the method is very time consuming and involves a great deal of physical effort for her because, with her particular condition, there is a great deal of involuntary movement whenever she tries to carry out a manual task. Just reaching out in order to grasp the joystick handle in the first place is, in itself, very difficult, with her hand and arm sometimes ‘overshooting’ the target. It isn't just hand movement that has this effect. Even if Claire just tries to speak, this also triggers off a range of involuntary movements and this, too, can be tiring for her.

In contrast, when there are no physical movement demands on Claire, she has learnt to sit reasonably still with comparatively little involuntary movement. Researchers in COGAIN have found indications that eye movement is not ‘connected’ to other voluntary body movements, and voluntary eye movement does not cause involuntary movements of the body in the same way as when trying to move a hand or arm, for example. This suggested that eye gaze may both allow communication for Claire, and also relieve her from her involuntary body movements caused by trying to manipulate a joystick, (Figure 8.3, left).

When eye tracking was tried with Claire, using an eye control system and experimental on-screen button software used by COGAIN, the results were encouraging. The system did manage to cope with a certain amount of involuntary head movement, whether forwards, backwards or sideways. When she tried eye-writing, despite the cognitive load of concentrating on eye-typing using an initially unfamiliar on-screen keyboard she still managed to remain comparatively still. Nonetheless, the targets had to remain reasonably large to maintain accuracy and communicate using an on-screen grid (Figure 8.3, right). Claire's successful typing already showed strong indications that eye control might have the potential to be both quicker and less tiring (because of the sharp reduction in involuntary head movement), and more comfortable for Claire.

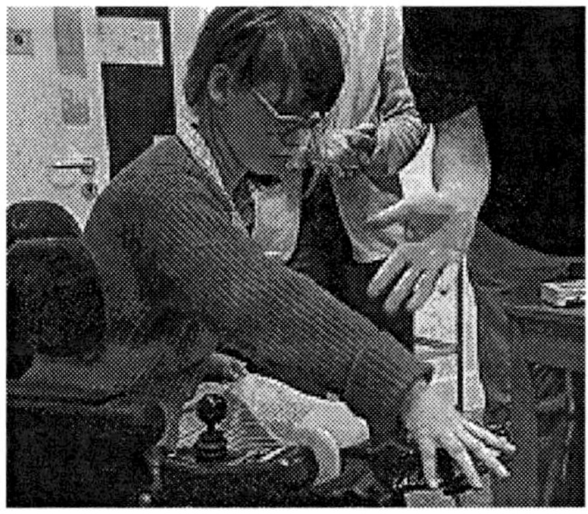
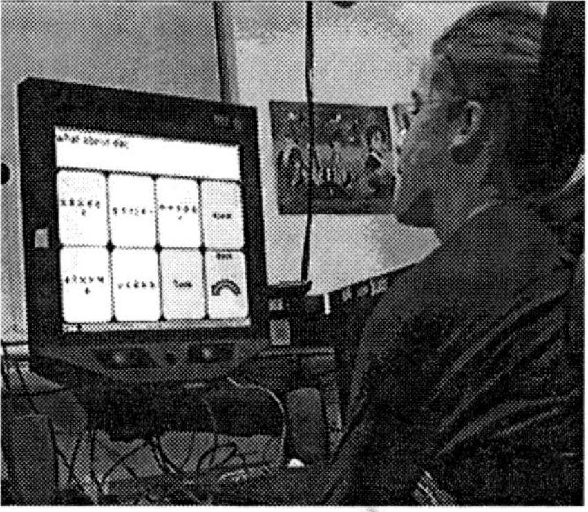

Figure 8.3. Claire using a wheelchair joystick, and using eye gaze to communicate

8.3.4 Michael

Michael is in his early 40's and has a wife and three boys. He had a severe stroke about 2 years ago and now, after rehabilitation, is back at home. He cannot speak but communicates by looking at letters on an 'e-tran frame' (Figure 8.4, left).

Before his stroke, Michael was very active and enjoyed a wide range of leisure pursuits. Despite the stroke, he remains a very intelligent man with an excellent sense of humour. He would like to be able to access his computer quickly and efficiently in order to communicate socially and assist with his wife's business. However, at present, his only form of access to technology is via switches. This he finds very slow and frustrating and he would very much like to use eye control as a quicker and easier method, if at all possible.

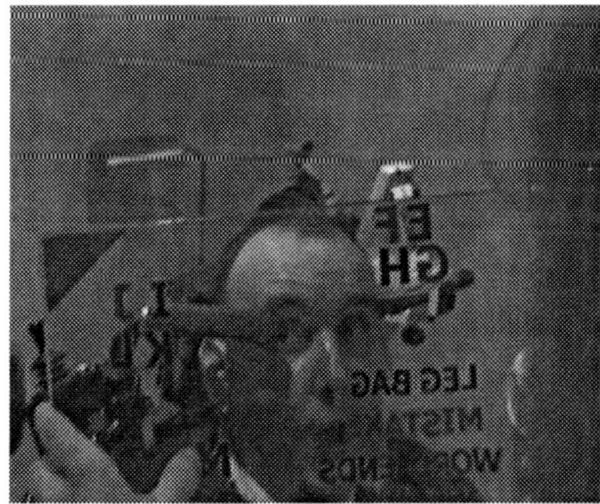
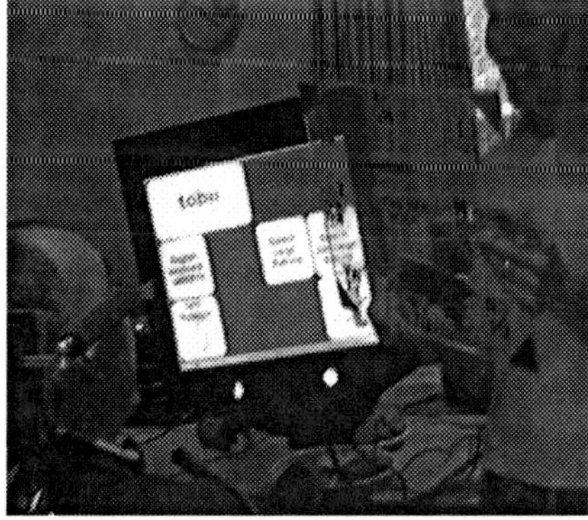

Figure 8.4. Michael using his e-tran frame, and using eye gaze, on-screen keys and the e-tran together to communicate

Because of the stroke, Michael has a certain amount of difficulty with head control. In addition, he has nystagmus, which means that he cannot fix his gaze in the same way that most other people can. Both of Michael's eyes have a significant amount of involuntary side-to-side movement (nystagmus) which tends to become more severe when he is tired.

Several eye tracking systems were tried with Michel, with little success due to his nystagmus. Finally, an advanced eye tracking system used within COGAIN was tried with him (Figure 8.4, right). With this particular system (Advanced Tobii system under development with COGAIN), if there are any specific areas of the screen that require re-calibration due to eye calibration drift or poor tracking, they can be selected and recalibrated individually. This presented a solution to his nystagmus. However, even if a successful calibration is achieved, account had to be taken of the fact that the nature of Michael's visual difficulties fluctuates and a successful calibration at one moment in time might not work effectively for him on another occasion.

On the occasions when Michael did achieve a successful calibration, the significant increase in speed that he was able to achieve in comparison with switches, combined with the greater comfort and satisfaction that the eye tracking system and software gave him, meant that he was extremely enthusiastic about eye control as an access method. His enthusiasm emphasised the importance of the need for developers within COGAIN to try to accommodate people like Michael by taking his kinds of access difficulties (involuntary head movement and fluctuating visual difficulties) into account.

8.4 What Can COGAIN Provide?

As illustrated by the case studies, COGAIN and its researchers operate by putting the needs of the end user first and foremost (Figure 8.5). The case studies clearly show that without their input and criticism we would be unable to design, produce and promote eye gaze systems that really work.

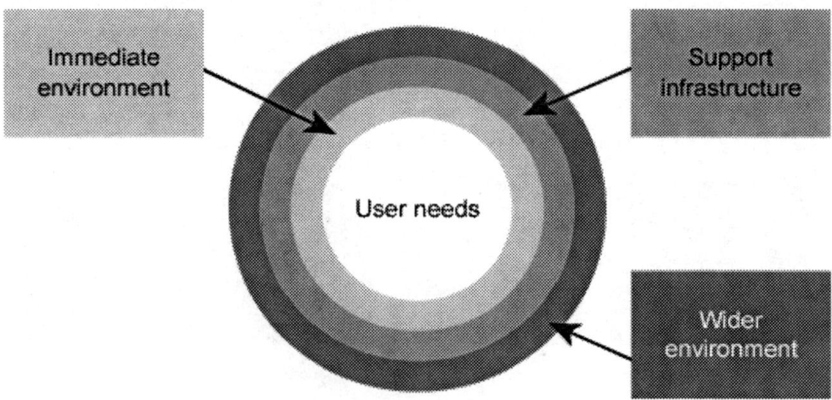

Figure 8.5. COGAIN places the needs of the end user first

COGAIN aims to provide a path to workable, practical and low-cost eye gaze communication. To help us achieve this COGAIN would like to encourage your participation, and in return we offer support *from* the network that is freely given in many areas including:

- Increased use of gaze driven technology in everyday life
- Development of very low-cost ubiquitous gaze trackers (Corno and Garbo, 2005)
- Reducing the cost of gaze systems and making them available to all
- Developing tools for rapid and natural text generation (typing, editing) (Aoki *et al.,* 2005)
- Developing gaze access and enabling solutions to existing technology
- Developing gaze aware and attentive interfaces (Hyrskykari *et al.,* 2005)
- Developing advanced gaze driven communication tools (text-to-speech systems, SMS generation, email access and generation, web access)
- Developing methods for using gaze to control personal environments to increase the autonomy of users (*e.g.* gaze driven home automation)
- Developing methods for using gaze to control personal mobility to increase the autonomy of users (*e.g.* gaze driven wheelchairs)
- For users with less severe impairments, providing a possibility for multiple modalities (*e.g.* gaze in combination with speech, or head pointing) (Elevesjo *et al.,* 2005)
- Developing gaze driven edutainment applications (such as games, shoot 'em up, crosswords, chess (Figure 8.6))
- Develop virtual environment gaze driven interfaces for research, natural interaction and edutainment applications (Bates *et al.,* 2005)
- Bringing together research teams, access providers, and end users in regular meetings and providing a platform for discussions and for knowledge sharing
- Making work user-driven.

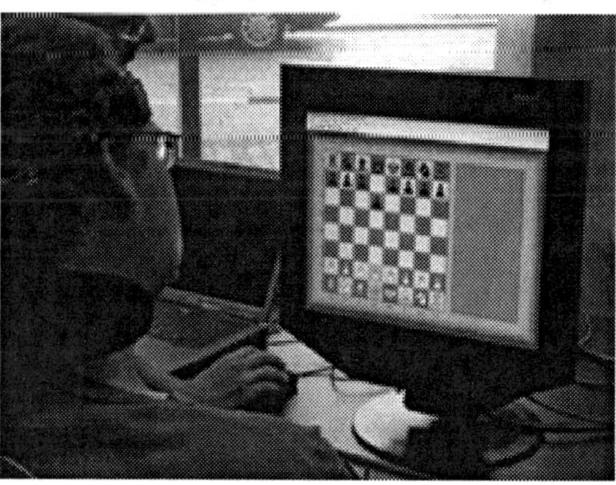

Figure 8.6. The COGAIN EyeChess program - playing chess by eye gaze alone

8.5 Summary

COGAIN aims to provide a path to practical and low-cost eye gaze communication and control in partnership with end users, workers in the field and researchers, so that we may work together to enable greater communication by eye gaze for high-level motor disabled users, so please get in touch with us at: – http://www.cogain.org/.

8.6 References

Aoki H, Itoh K, Hansen JP (2005) Learning to type Japanese text by Gaze Interaction in six hours. In: Proceedings of HCI International 2005, Las Vegas, USA

Bates R, Istance HO, Donegan M, Oosthuizen L (2005) Fly where you look: enhancing gaze based interaction in 3D environments. In: Proceedings of HCI International 2005, Las Vegas, USA

Corno F, Garbo A (2005) Multiple low-cost cameras for effective head and gaze tracking. In: Proceedings of HCI International 2005, Las Vegas, USA

Elevesjo J, Hansen DW, Hansen JP, Johansen AS (2005) Mainstreaming gaze interaction towards a mass market for the benefit of all. In: Proceedings of HCI International 2005, Las Vegas, USA

Hyrskykari A, Majaranta P, Räihä K-J (2005) From gaze control to attentive interfaces. In: Proceedings of HCI International 2005, Las Vegas, USA

Jordansen IK, Boedeker S, Donegan M, Oosthuizen L, di Girolamo M *et al.* (2005) D7.2 report on a market study and demographics of user population. Communication by Gaze Interaction (COGAIN), IST-2003-511598: Deliverable 7.2. Available at: http://www.cogain.org/results/reports/COGAIN-D7.2.pdf

Chapter 9

Older Users' Requirements for Interactive Television

H. Boyle, C. Nicolle, M. Maguire and V. Mitchell

9.1 Introduction

In Britain some 62% of households have access to digital television, and the British government has mapped out a plan to steadily shut down all analogue TV signals by 2012 (Lowery Miller, 2005), with the expectation that all UK households will benefit from the digital future. Over the next few years, television and the Internet are expected to converge even more to create a communication and information medium for the mass market, enabling on-line access without the need to purchase and learn the intricacies of computers.

With digital technology being actively encouraged by the Government, how can interactive television (iTV) in the future be designed to improve the lives of older people? And which services will be of particular benefit to them? Older people often have a combination of impairments such as poor hearing/vision, reduced mobility/ dexterity, and may have reduced cognitive ability. Zajicek (2001) states that the ageing process affects an individual's ability to function successfully with the standard graphical user interface and that the capabilities required for interaction with an interface are the ones that deteriorate most markedly with age. However, older people are generally willing to use computers and find the experience a satisfying one. Older computer users are an important group from whom to ascertain if there is an interest in the uptake of iTV. But equally, is there the same interest in uptake by older non-computer users? Most importantly, what are the user requirements from both computer and non-computer older users that must be met to provide an inclusive iTV service?

Keates and Clarkson (2004) identified specific causes for concern with regard to interaction with digital television (DTV) using a set top box (STB). The majority of their sample ranged from 62-85 years old, and they found that for this population there was a high cognitive, visual and dexterity demand from use of the DTV. They recommended to manufacturers that cognitive demand should be kept to a minimum and the interaction with the STBs should be as transparent as possible. This, they advocate, is not aimed just at a small section of the market, but instead is good design for everyone.

Organisations that are promoting iTV should consider older users' requirements to facilitate maximum independence, both in their usage of the system and in the activities of daily living. To make this happen, there must be sufficient interest and action from service providers to promote the inclusive design concept. This study is therefore a step forward in attempting to identify what older users' requirements are for the future of inclusive iTV.

9.2 Background

This study was undertaken in part-fulfilment of the requirements for the postgraduate course in Ergonomics at Loughborough University. The objective was to evaluate what older users' requirements are for iTV, including the services that they would value (*e.g.*, e-mail or the World Wide Web), and explore barriers (*e.g.*, technology complexity, usability, *etc.*). This was part of a larger project, the Services Aggregation Project (SA), part of The Application Home Initiative (TAHI at http://www.theapplicationhome.com), undertaken at the Ergonomics and Safety Research Institute and sponsored by the Department of Trade and Industry. Under the auspices of Severn Trent Water and with the support of Leicester City Council, an energy and water efficiency monitoring trial (called SMART) was installed within a number of homes in Leicestershire as a pilot study. The trial was developed to build upon an Automatic Meter Reading System, which would feed a server-based system, an XTN hub from Extrada, which would then aggregate the metering data with water and energy saving advice and other services, to provide an aggregated services set. The trial utilised Digital TV set top boxes in each trial home, enabling both email and web browsing. To augment this service and to encourage the user to look at the water and energy consumption data, a number of other services were also provided, including saving advice, home shopping, entertainment and meal planning (see Figure 9.1). These services had been re-purposed for TV format and were accessible from an Internet portal via the TV and digital Netgem box. Overall the TAHI SA project had three objectives:

- to test user reactions to the SMART set of services;
- to test the usability of the services and learn lessons for future design;
- to study user acceptance of the idea of receiving services through a TV (as opposed to a PC).

In addition, the project was interested in targeting structured groups of older users to assist in formulating and promoting future iTV applications. As older people are the fastest growing sector in the world's population, the issue of accessibility and usability of these products and services has become critical. Since a very large percentage of the television audience, especially during the daytime and non-peak viewing hours, is made up of disabled and elderly people (Gill, 2004), it is clear that service providers should give more thought to providing more inclusive access.

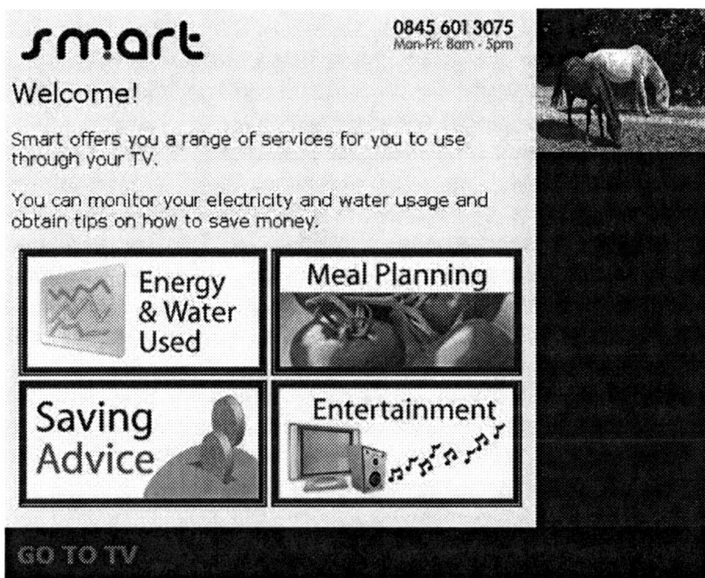

Figure 9.1. SMART home page

This is where the current study began, and where the University of the Third Age (U3A) came on board (although we have to say that our users from U3A were certainly not the 'stay at home' type!). Although the usability of iTV in this specific part of the project was not under investigation (for the usability assessment see Maguire *et al.,* 2005), it was essential to assess its usability to some extent in order to understand the older users' requirements. The focus therefore was to:

- identify user requirements for iTV services concerning older users;
- address concerns/barriers that would need to be overcome;
- formulate recommendations for future successful implementation of iTV in older users' homes.

9.3 Methodology

Data collection of user requirements involved qualitative research methods over two phases. The first phase consisted of three focus groups with a total of twenty participants, taking place in June 2005. This method was chosen because focus groups offered an efficient way to provide qualitative user feedback on the Interactive TV services being considered. Although a survey could have been conducted with a wider range of people, it was felt that this would not produce the same richness of data and allow users to refine their views in discussion with others. The groups were made up of computer and non-computer users from local groups of the University of the Third Age. A married couple from the U3A offered their home for the first focus group and the user trials, in order to provide a realistic environment to maximise the potential of iTV. SMART was installed in their home, including the energy and water usage monitoring system, but due to budget constraints STBs could not be offered to all participants, at least at this stage. The other two focus groups were held at ESRI.

The basic procedure was as follows: For each group, the iTV and the SMART system were demonstrated. The users were then asked to discuss their initial requirements, concerns and issues related to the service. A concept board was then introduced to generate new concepts and ideas on iTV. The participants were encouraged to select pictures from a range provided and then to choose an image that would represent facilities they would like to see on iTV. Using a word map, participants were also asked to provide a word or sentence on their concerns or issues, and these were placed on a flip chart to prompt further discussion.

The second phase of the study involved user trials with eight participants from the first focus group. Performing user-based testing allowed the users to experience the TV services and rate their usefulness while also indicating to the evaluator how usable the services were. The aims of the user trials were:

- to reinforce the function of the iTV;
- to allow the participants to experience iTV;
- to explore the findings from the focus group even further in order to highlight the key user requirements, concerns/barriers/issues, *etc.*;
- to identify if there are any differences between computer/non-computer users;
- to rate the equipment and services on an individual basis;
- to identify participants' impairments further to ascertain if there are any problems in interacting with the iTV.

The participants carried out a pre-defined set of usage scenarios using the iTV. The tasks given to the users involved: viewing and interpreting energy and water usage charts on the TV screen, planning a meal with certain ingredients using the Cheffy meal planning tool, identifying energy and water saving tips, finding famous quotes online, performing a Google search, and sending an email using the digital TV email service.

User interface issues and user ratings of the different services were recorded. These tasks were followed by a semi-structured interview to provide further detailed information on user requirements. User ratings of the services indicated that the most popular were TV-based Internet and email, as well as advice on saving energy and water.

One might question whether older people from U3A are representative of the older population in general. These participants ranged from lecturers, teachers, doctors, to engineers, *etc.*, coming from similar socio-economic backgrounds, and hence their views may differ from those of other older people. In addition 15 out of 20 of them were computer users. However, the sample can be justified as the service provider sought to target structured groups of older people such as the U3A to use as a platform, *i.e.*, it has transfer potential. Further trials are, however, recommended to cover a wider range of older users from different educational and social groups. The sample for both the focus groups and user trials is provided in Tables 9.1 and 9.2 below:

Table 9.1. Focus groups sample (total 20)

Gender		**Age**		**Computer Usage**	
Males	8	80-89 yrs	2	Computer users	15
Females	12	70-79 yrs	16	Non-computer users	5
		60-69 yrs	2		

Table 9.2. User trials sample (total 8)

Gender		**Age**	**Computer Usage**	
Males	4	From 73 to 86	Computer users	4
Females	4		Non-computer users	4

9.4 Analysis and Results

9.4.1 Main Themes of User Requirements

A thematic approach to data analysis was used including three steps: data reduction, data display and conclusion drawing/verification (Hignett, 2004). The data from both the focus groups and user trials were transcribed and imported into a qualitative data management tool, Nvivo (http://www.qsrinternational.com/). The data were summarised and coded to identify key themes and their sub-categories, and memos, quotes, and references were linked to codes where relevant.

Emergent patterns were selected according to how many times a specific point was mentioned in the data. 14 main themes were identified, with codes being added, removed or relocated to reflect additional data and iterative analysis. Each main theme was then decomposed, in both diagrammatic and tabular form, into its sub-codes. Six of these main themes are headings for the services provided by SMART (*e.g.*, energy and usage, saving tips, *etc.*), with the users rating those services. The remaining eight (requirements, concerns, impairments, iTV, computers, equipment, U3A, e-mail) are the themes that were identified from the conceptual framework of knowledge and comments at the start of a project. It is important to note, however, that although user requirements had a separate heading within Nvivo, specific requirements overlapped with the other themes. The 14 key themes/trees from the data collection were then systematically re-coded in order to identify prominent patterns, which were then used as a framework to investigate all the results from the focus groups and user trials (see the data display in Figure 9.2).

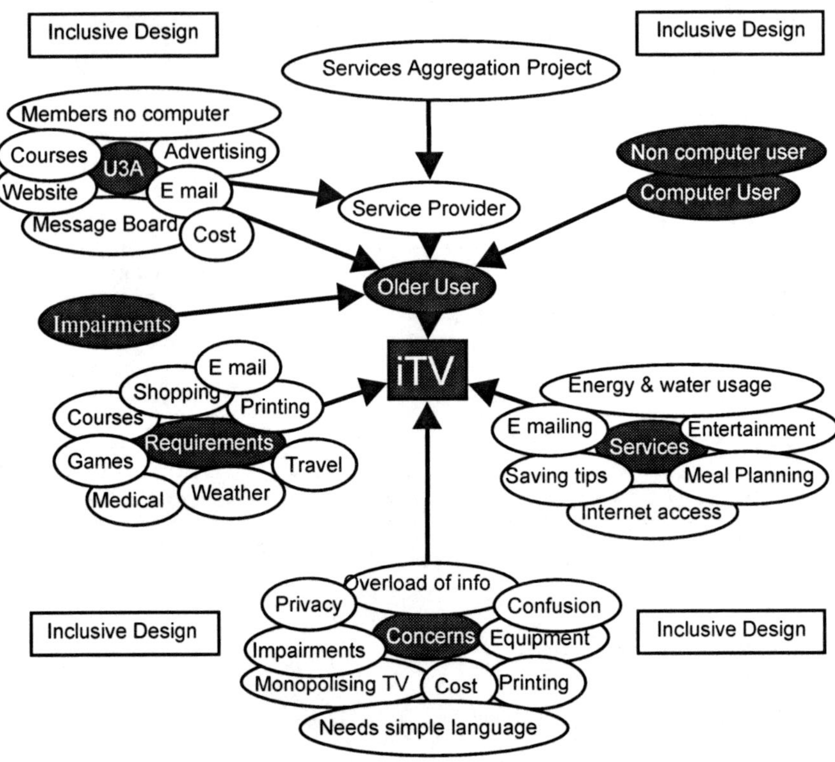

Figure 9.2. Data display as a framework for analysis

9.4.2 iTV Concerns

To illustrate with just one example from the main themes, there were 28 sub-codes in total under the theme 'Concerns,' from which nine key concerns were extracted (see bottom of Figure 9.2). These highlighted the main issues or barriers that older users may have: overload of information (TV was for relaxation and not for looking up information), privacy (if other family members are present when using email), confusion (iTV offers more functionality and thus requires more cognitive effort to learn and operate than ordinary TV), equipment (some usability issues with the remote control and the need for wrist support when using the keyboard on one's lap), printing (facility not available), monopolising the TV (when others may wish to watch it), cost (of the STB, broadband, and services), impairments (*e.g.*, difficulties manipulating the remote control due to arthritis, and difficulties scanning the TV and reading the keyboard when wearing varifocals or separate glasses for reading and distance), and the need for simple language.

Since the sample of users was relatively well educated and articulate (U3A), with a large proportion having computer experience, it is likely that many of these concerns would be amplified for many other older people. These themes provide useful context for the design of iTV services in the future.

9.5 Conclusions and Recommendations

In summary, this study found that computer users and non-computer users were positive about iTV. However, computer users were a bit more apprehensive due to the lack of privacy, printing, sending of attachments and access to Word, *etc.*, but this did not seem to be an issue with non-computer users. A number of impairments (including difficulties with vision, hearing and dexterity) limited access to the iTV when using the keyboard or remote control and when viewing the interface. Concerns and barriers need to be addressed to accommodate older users' requirements. Cost, overload of information, confusion regarding the technology, the need for simple navigation/language, and the design of the remote control and keyboard for iTV use are all such areas that need to be targeted. It seems that this group of older users would be willing to use the iTV in the future if (1) the benefits are clear to them, (2) they receive adequate instruction, and (3) the system itself is easy to use.

The project has made a number of recommendations to ensure a more inclusive design of iTV which will meet older users' requirements, for example:

- in order to accommodate users with visual impairments and limited dexterity, ensure that relevant design guidelines are adhered to (*e.g.*, from CENELEC at www.cenelec.org/Cenelec/Homepage.htm, the BBC at www.bbc.co.uk/commissioning/bbci/pdf/styleguide2_1.pdf, the RNIB and COST 219ter at www.tiresias.org/cost219ter/about.htm and www.tiresias.org/guidelines/television.htm);
- to reduce wrist, back or neck strain, consider innovative hardware design solutions, *e.g.*, a keyboard offering more stability and comfort on the lap, perhaps with a gel/sponge base;
- install the set top box at an appropriate height to allow for ease of access (three out of the eight in the user trials had problems with their knees and hips);
- to reduce overload of information, consider personalised information services for specific users or groups of users;
- provide the ability to communicate with other key people in the community, *e.g.* doctors, nurses, advisors, and any other services users require;
- provide the facility to send attachments, print and access Word;
- enhance communication and entertainment services;
- enable customisation of the interface design (layout, text size, contrast, *etc.*);
- promote and facilitate the re-purposing of websites and services for iTV viewing;

- incorporate a help line into the service provision to reduce anxiety, especially by older users. Although TV digital services such as Freeview do not normally provide such help, this might be an opportunity for digibox manufacturers to make their products more attractive. Electrical stores competing on the high street are also realising the benefit of providing more technical help to customers;
- provide a clear breakdown of costs, *e.g.*, broadband, equipment, services, support, *etc.*, which is paramount in attracting older users.

This study suggests that for the time being, for older users, the main focus for iTV applications should be on entertainment and simple communication. The common need for entertainment is the predominant driving force behind the traditional TV, and interactivity seems to be foreign to the traditional use of TV for at least some older users. As one participant mentioned, she does not want to be bombarded with information when sitting in front of a TV – she is in the mode of escaping and relaxing. However, this may change with the next older generation, who will be used to information "on tap" through multi-modal interaction devices. This project has covered only a small sample of older users and highlighted certain requirements and issues. In order to ascertain a global overview of older people's requirements, a more lengthy study is required, including a wider range of older users with different backgrounds and experiences in the use of technology.

9.6 References

Gill J (2004) Inclusive design of interactive television. Available at: http://www.tiresias.org /reports/dtg.htm

Hignett S (2004) Qualitative methodology. In: Wilson JR, Corlett N (eds.) Evaluation of human work, 3rd edn. Taylor and Francis, London, UK

Keates S, Clarkson J (2004) Assessing the accessibility of digital television set-top boxes. In: Keates S *et al.* (eds.) Designing a more inclusive world. Springer, London, UK

Lowery Miller K (2005) The airwaves go digital. Newsweek (6–13 June): 59–63

Maguire M, Mitchell V, Nicolle C (2005) TAHI services aggregation project, SMART service development and user trial. Ergonomics and Safety Research Institute, Loughborough University, UK

Zajicek M (2001) Supporting older adults at the interface. In: Proceedings of the Interact 2001, Tokyo, Japan

Chapter 10

InclusiveCAD: A Software Resource for Designers

A.S. Macdonald, D. Loudon, P.J. Rowe, D. Samuel, V. Hood, A.C. Nicol and B. Conway

10.1 Introduction

The functional demand placed on older adults during the normal activities of daily living is of concern to a number of health professionals and designers, as well as the clients and their carers. This paper reports on the endeavour to produce a first generation model of the human subject in motion performing a range of daily tasks, and to convey complex biomechanical function related movement and strength data in a simple, understandable, scientific and analytical manner, appropriate for use by designers in a CAD environment. The changing level of demand placed on the joint is conveyed by a variable colour sphere located at the joint which changes from green through yellow and orange to red corresponding to increasing levels of demand. Early feedback indicates that although primarily intended for designers, the tool has value to a broader range of stakeholders, also including health professionals and carers.

This paper reports on the EPSRC EQUAL-funded project GR/R26856/01, researched jointly by the Bioengineering Unit at the University of Strathclyde in Glasgow, the School of Health Sciences at Queen Margaret University College in Edinburgh, and Product Design Engineering at The Glasgow School of Art.

For a designer to develop a product specification, and ultimately to embody into a product solution, features and qualities appropriate to the end user, s/he must synthesise many different types and qualities of information. For the inclusive designer, it is vital to consider information on user capability. However, to date, there has been very limited information available about the functional demand placed on individuals when performing daily tasks or interacting with products. Understanding of functional demand is of particular importance in the case of designing for older people to ensure that products are usable and match capability without causing injury.

In addition to the general lack of information, any information that is available is too often presented in a format that is at best onerous to use, at worst incomprehensible, and fails to recognise the needs of the designer or the processes of design. As the interaction between people, products and environments is a dynamic process, the typically static representation of information in statistical tabulation formats proves of questionable value to a designer. There is a real risk of misapplying what information is available, which at present requires specialist knowledge, interpretation and calculation. Current information sources also tend to ignore the environment within, and the tools with which designers work, particularly the predominant use of CAD software in the design process.

10.2 Methods

In the University of Strathclyde's BioEngineering Unit, data was obtained on the functional demands of a set of five defined activities of daily living, using a sample group of 84 older male and female participants in the age groups 60s, 70s and 80+. Isometric strength data was measured using a purpose-built dynamometer and biomechanical functional movement data recorded with a VICON 8-camera motion analysis system with three Kistler forceplates (Figure 10.1). Activities consisted of gait, sit-stand-sit, door opening and closing, stair ascent and descent, and lifting a small object to different heights. VICON BodyBuilder was used to analyse the data, calculate joint angles and moments and export limb segment positions as a series of rotations and translations from the position of the pelvis segment (Figure 10.2) (Rowe *et al.*, 2005).

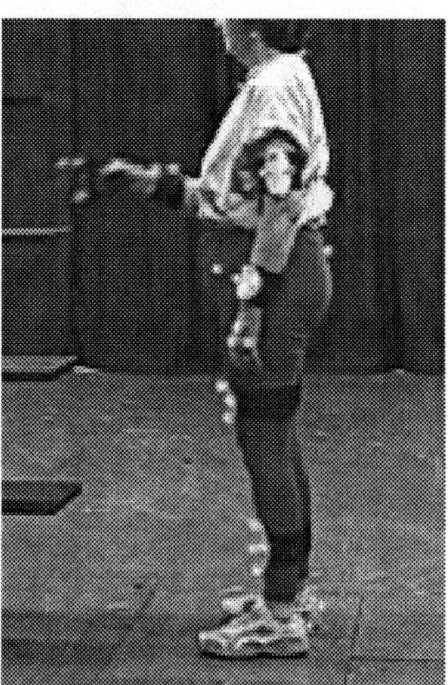

Figure 10.1. Data being collected during a functional task

The researchers proposed that this data would be of great value to designers if it could be made usable and accessible. However, numerical data or graphs of joint moments, joint angles and functional demand data was found to require skill in interpretation and a level of biomechanical comprehension and training beyond most of the community which the researchers wished to reach, involve and educate – particularly designers, and even if there was a level of comprehension, it was still time consuming to interpret the data.

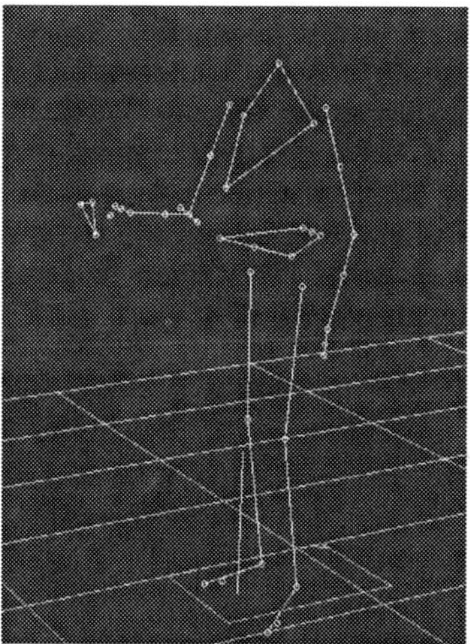

Figure 10.2. Data collected during a functional task processed in Vicon BodyBuilder

For these reasons the movement of the subject during the activity was reanimated. This was achieved by the creation of a software application, implemented in Visual C++ and OpenGL, which displayed real-time generated 3D animated visualisations of participants performing the activities. The animated human model consisted of simple cylindrical or block representations of the body segments from the VICON model rendered frame by frame in three dimensions in light blue. The hands were displayed as 3D hand models shaded as flesh tone. The real-time animation showed the subject performing the functional task in a realistic way. In order to express the functional demand visually, each segment was connected to the next segment by a node representing the joint as a variable-colour sphere. Functional demand – calculated as the external moment expressed as a percentage of the maximum available isometric strength available at the joint at that angle – was represented on a continuous colour gradient from green through yellow to red. A green colour was shown where functional demand was below 40%. Where the functional demand for that joint was higher but still within acceptable limits (between 40% and 80%) the sphere turned from green to yellow to orange. Finally, if the joint was experiencing functional demand levels deemed to be unacceptable (above 80%), the sphere turned red. This 'traffic light' system was thought to be a clear and immediate way of allowing the designer to understand, without specialist knowledge, the functional demands placed on individuals while performing daily activities, and at the same time to allow designers to understand the design implications of product and environmental concepts developed in response to need.

The software was integrated with the engineering CAD package SolidWorks, a popular tool with product designers, implemented as a plug-in in C++, using the Solidworks Application Interface (Figure 10.3). This enabled a virtual model of a product to be imported and attached to the hand of the human model, and the effects of the product weight on the arm joints calculated. The arm of the human model could be manipulated by moving the hand with the mouse pointer, and the arm position resolved using inverse kinematics. Hence, it was possible to evaluate the effects of different upper limb configurations and objects held in the hand on the moments generated during the functional task. The effects of varying the parameters of the CAD model are calculated quickly and immediately visualised. For the example of a jug kettle, parameters such as the shape of a kettle, material properties, handle position and orientation, and water fill level can be varied and immediate feedback is given of the change in demands that the design of a particular kettle places on the older adult (Figure 10.4).

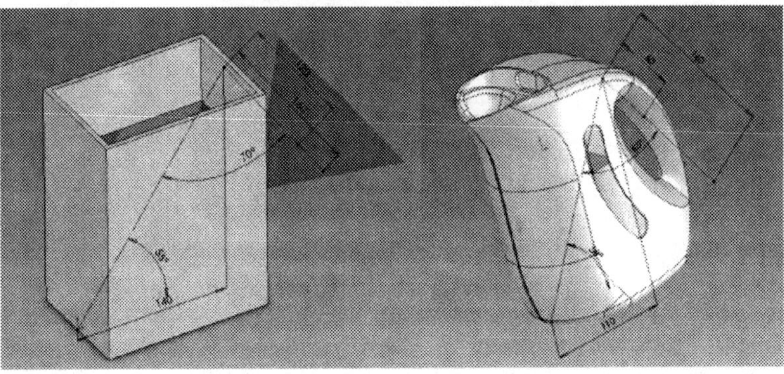

Figure 10.3. CAD models of a stereotypical kettle imported from Solidworks

10.3 Discussion

Envisioning functional demand in this way was shown to be effective in reducing the need for specialist knowledge. This is achieved by combining moment data, angle data, the direction of moment (flexion/extension), and angle varying muscle strength, and simply expressing it as 'how hard the muscles are working as a percentage of their maximum capability' through the 'traffic light' method. This is something which the layman can understand, and provides a medium for the communication of important results of biomechanical analysis to those beyond the boundary of the biomechanics knowledge domain.

The choice of visual representation method allows the functional demand of tasks of everyday living to be communicated in a form which can be immediately appreciated and understood across all interested parties, with potential applications in both design and healthcare. Initial feedback has been encouraging. This was evident from a demonstration of the prototype tool to all the main stakeholders: the various healthcare professionals, bio-engineers, designers, and the subjects (older adults) themselves. For example, a designer can quickly understand the effect of the weight of an object whereas a physiotherapist can quickly understand how much load should be tolerated during exercise.

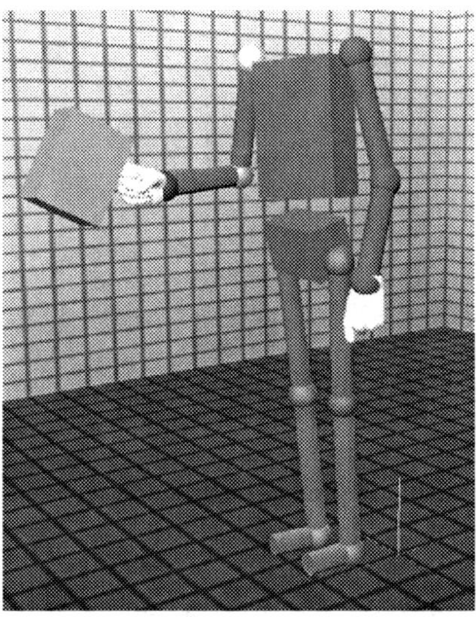

Figure 10.4. Visual C++ model showing body segments and traffic light system for joint functional demand

As the animations of the individuals performing the tasks are from motion capture, the motions have a 'life-like' quality. There are differences, often subtle, in the way that different individuals perform the same motion, which have a corresponding effect on the stresses at the joints (Figures 10.5 and 10.6). If the tool is to be viable, this highlights the need for sufficient complete data sets.

An interesting outcome of the prototype tool is that the viewer gets a glimpse into the experience of the user. This qualitative aspect of the tool will be explored further, with the potential of being used in the early stages of design, where freehand sketches are often used in preference to CAD modelling.

This first generation prototype of the biomechanical interaction of a virtually modelled product with the upper limbs of the virtual human model has shown its potential as a means of assessing the demands that a product concept's attributes (*e.g.*, weight, centre of mass, handle position) places on users. The integration of the tool with CAD software enables the designer to obtain feedback quickly, encouraging several iterations of analysis during the design process.

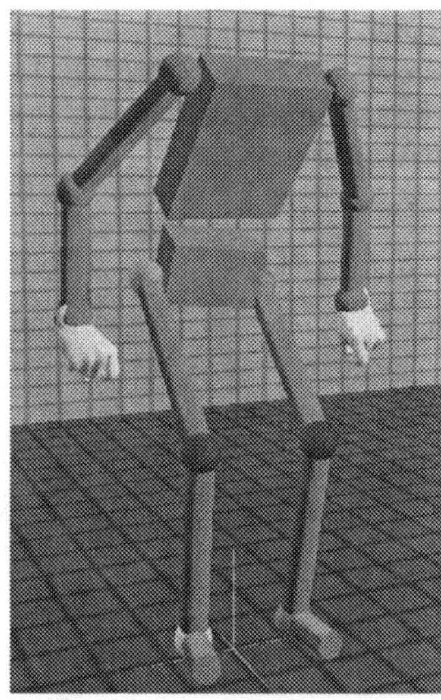

Figure 10.5. The functional demand on the lower limbs while rising to stand

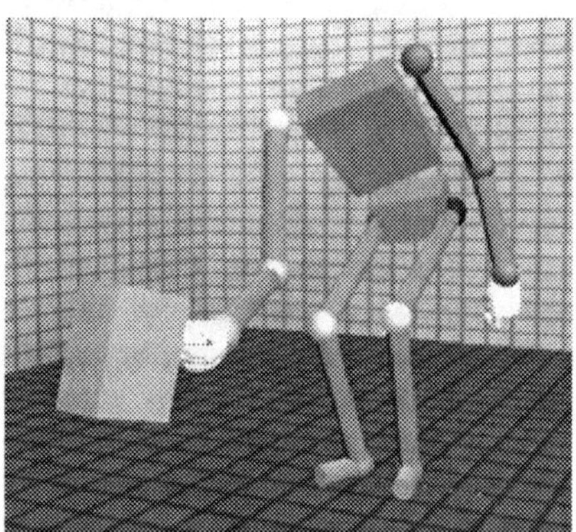

Figure 10.6. The functional demand on the upper and lower limbs when reaching while rising

Having produced a first generation proof-of-concept, the next stage is seen as its careful and systematic evaluation by all the stakeholders – bioengineers, designers, health scientists, health and social care providers, older adults and their carers, and human factors experts. Already, in discussions with biomechanics researchers, several guidelines and 'rules of thumb' have been identified that would be of value to designers when considering the limitations of older users. Integrating these guidelines into the tool will give further context and explanation of what is happening in these movements during everyday tasks. A good analogy here is the work by Pirkl (1994), which describes the physical changes in capability of the senses and motor movements with age, the functional effect, the problems this causes and how, *e.g.*, these are interpreted into a series of strategies and guidelines for designers to allow them to determine the design characteristics of potential solutions for products, interfaces and environments that are able to safely accommodate the functional limitations of older users.

Although originally intended as a tool for designers, the feedback and evaluation of this method of visualising the data is beginning to suggest that this tool may be of value across all those involved in professional caring for older adults.

10.4 References

Loudon D, Macdonald AS (2004) Virtual design verification for inclusive design through software. In: Proceedings of CWUAAT'04, Cambridge, UK

Loudon D, Macdonald AS (2005) Software tool for designers. In: Proceedings of INCLUDE 2005, Royal College of Art, London, UK

Pirkl JJ, Babic, AL (1988) Guidelines and strategies for designing transgenerational products: a resource manual for industrial design professionals. Acton, MA, USA

Rowe PJ, Hood V, Loudon D, Samuel D, Nicol AC *et al.* (2005) Calculating and presenting biomechanical functional demand in older adults during activities of daily living. In: Proceedings of the IASTED BioMech2005, Benidorm, Spain

Chapter 11

Towards an Interactive System Eliciting Narrative Comprehension in Children with Autism: A Longitudinal Study

M. Davis, K. Dautenhahn, C. Nehaniv and S. Powell

11.1 Introduction

Research has shown a deficit in the comprehension and creation of narrative in children with autism which impacts on their social skills. Children with autism form a very diverse group; our research agenda is to develop an interactive software system that elicits children's narrative comprehension while addressing the needs of *individual* children. This chapter documents progress towards an adaptive interactive software system (in the context of a game) for children with autism, specifically in the context of narrative and social understanding, and presents results from a longitudinal study involving 12 children. The work falls under the umbrella of the Aurora project (Aurora, 2000) which, through focussed studies, investigates the potential enhancement of the everyday lives of children with autism through the use of robots and other interactive systems as therapeutic or educational 'toys'. A playful context and enjoyment are central to our approach.

11.2 Autism, Narrative and Social Comprehension

Autism is a lifelong pervasive developmental disorder affecting social ability. Although people with autism form a very diverse group, they all exhibit impaired social interaction and communication, and have a limited range of imaginative activities, collectively referred to as the *triad of impairments* (Frith, 1989; Wing 1996; Powell, 1999). Additionally it is common to find particular sensitivities (Bogdashina, 2003), repetitive behaviour patterns and resistance to change in routine (NAS, 2004). People with autism have great difficulty making sense of the world, in particular the social world. We do not imply that there is no meaning to the lives of people with autism, but that socially constructed meaning is difficult.

The more socially constructed the meaning, the greater the difficulty. Autobiographical accounts such as Grandin (1995) show that people with autism who do live successfully in the, to them bizarre, world of so-called 'normal people' do so at least in part by learning explicit rules: for example, remember to look interested when someone is talking to you; or, if someone smiles at you, you should smile back (note that even this apparently simple rule does not always apply).

It is postulated that narrative is central to the construction of social meaning. By fitting events into a narrative pattern we construct and inhabit a meaningful, consistent and predictable world (Bruner, 1986, 1990, 2002; Schank, 1990; Linde, 1993). We develop our sense of self and are able to understand the behaviours of others (people or other agents which we imbue with intent), and to respond in ways seen as meaningful and consistent. Narrative gives a framework for interpreting new events, in particular surprising events or behaviours which do not accord with our expectations, and for fitting them into a temporal framework (Schank, 1990; Bruner, 2002; Porter Abbott, 2002).

It has been shown that children with autism do have some specific difficulties with narrative. Studies using narrative pictures showed references to causality and affect may be missing or inappropriate (Tager-Flushberg and Sullivan, 1995; Capps *et al.,* 2000). Abell *et al.* (2000) showed, using animated triangles, that children with autism were more likely to attribute inappropriate mental states than typically developing children or those with general intellectual impairment. This impairment in mentalising is often attributed to a deficit in a theory of mind (Baron-Cohen, 1999). However, narrative comprehension may be viewed as causal rather than symptomatic; as being fundamental to the perception, creation and communication of meaning in social interaction (Bruner and Feldman, 1993; Dautenhahn, 2002; Hutto, 2003). Thus we may view difficulties with narrative as underlying the social and temporal difficulties we see in autism.

There are a number of theories of narrative comprehension, but it is clear that each narratee actively constructs an internal representation of the narrative, sometimes called a *situation model.* The constructionist theory (Graesser and Wienner-Hastings, 1999) predicts that the narratee will make inferences which establish both local and global *coherence*, and *explain* events and motivations. Picture narratives are of particular interest to us; in the domain of comics McCloud (1993) refers to our ability to construct a continuous situation model, *'mentally construct a continuous, unified reality',* from discrete panels. He refers to the space between the panels as central, *'the very heart of comics'.*

What then is narrative? Views vary widely: we are concerned here with simple narratives in which the chronology of the exposition follows the chronology of events in the story; and in which the story follows, or is a simple variation on, a format proposed by Bruner for a "story worth telling" (Bruner, 1986; Dautenhahn, 2002). This format supposes a sequence of events involving purposeful characters. The basic pattern of events comprises: a *steady state* which establishes a world view; a *precipitating event* which is some break in the steady state, unexpected by the protagonists, not necessarily by the audience; a *restoration* in which the precipitating event is resolved and some steady state restored; and a *coda* which signals that the narrative is at an end. Variations may occur on this skeleton; one narrative may nest inside another or a stage may be repeated, vestigial or merely assumed.

Relevant work exists in the area of software systems which elicit narrative from children such as Cassell's (2002) story listening systems, the PETS storyteller (Montemayor *et al.*, 2000), and the emergent narrative systems described by Aylett and Louchart (2003). Work with children with autism, in addition to the Aurora project previously mentioned, includes work in the area of educational games for children with autism (Sehaba *et al.*, 2005), and studies investigating the use of virtual reality systems with children with autism (Heerera and Veera, 2005; Moore *et al.*, 2005). Grynszpan (2005) is working towards guidelines for developing software for children with autism. Our work differs from these in that we are following individual children through a longitudinal study, focussing on 'primitive' elements of narrative, presented as proto-narratives, in an interactive adaptive software game.

11.3 The Preliminary Study

Our goal is to identify aspects of narrative where therapeutic intervention with interactive computer systems could be applied for individual children with autism. As we are concerned with narrative comprehension rather than ability to read we initially propose a software system which allows exploration of the abilities of children with autism to build coherent narratives from discrete stimuli such as events in pictures or photographs. Many children with autism have difficulties in understanding remote object references, such as pointing with a finger, and in generalization from one context to another. They may not understand how a mouse works, or may take a long time to learn, and so the software system was presented using a touch sensitive screen.

Children with autism form a heterogeneous group, a program or set of stories appropriate for one child will not necessarily be appropriate for another. As autistic subjects have difficulties with social interaction and communication, and may have limited productive language, usual methods of requirement elicitation and software evaluation, such as interviews, focus groups and collaborative design, are not possible. Therefore a pilot study was carried out using a simple fill-the-gap picture story activity concerned with narrative recognition and construction. In order to create a playful context the activity was presented as a 'game'; a playful task involving the experimenter and child. The study compared a physical game using laminated cards with a computer based version of the same game which we called TouchStory (see Figure 11.1.). A correct answer was rewarded with verbal praise, and in the case of TouchStory the on screen reward was that the remaining possible answers were removed, leaving just the complete story. In the case of a wrong answer the child was invited to try again. 18 children were involved and our intention was to investigate whether they were as engaged and successful with a touch sensitive screen as they were with physical cards. Results were encouraging (Davis *et al.*, 2004) and led to the preparation of a longitudinal study focussing in more depth on the particular aspects of narrative which individual children found difficult. The longitudinal study also uses an *adaptive phase* where the stories presented by the system varied depending on the *interaction history* with a particular child, *i.e.* the scores that child had achieved previously. The goal of this adaptation was to tailor the system towards the children's individual needs, aiming to provide more opportunities for learning in areas the children had difficulties, while still providing sufficient, rewarding experience in a play (game) context.

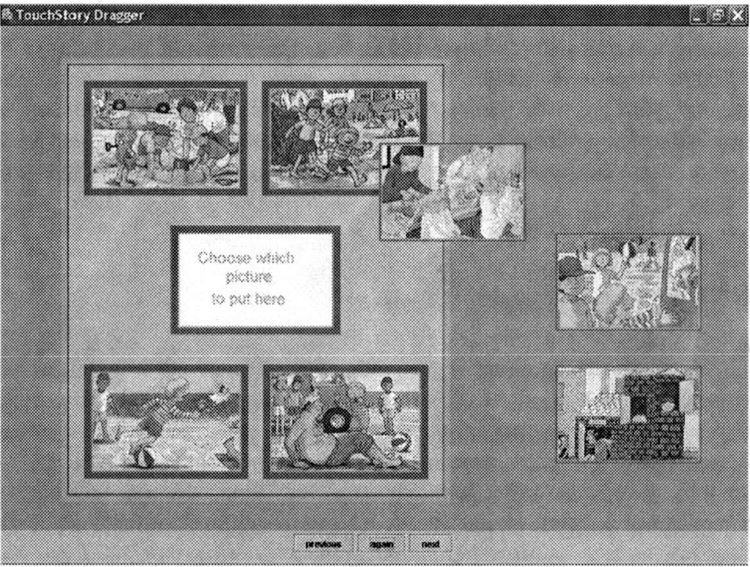

Figure 11.1. TouchStory in use during the prototype trials. Illustrations by Alex Brychta from The Hair Cut and The Big Box, by Rod Hunt, illustrated by Alex Brychta (Oxford Reading Tree, 1991), and from The Ice Cream, by Rod Hunt, illustrated by Alex Brychta (Oxford Reading Tree, 2003), copyright © Oxford University Press, reprinted by permission of Oxford University Press.

11.4 The Longitudinal Study

We introduce the term *t-story* to mean picture narratives and proto-narratives collectively, in contrast to the fully developed complex 'stories' of daily life. Our intention was to investigate 'primitive' elements of narrative (proto-narratives) as a precursor of narrative comprehension, using t-stories. Primitive elements of narrative were identified and t-stories prepared for each primitive type. The classification and an example from each type can be seen in Figures 11.2–11.7.

The longitudinal study used a set of 56 t-stories moderated for correctness and lack of ambiguity by a panel of 10 adults. The panel consisted of 7 men and 3 women, with a range of technical experience in using computers. The panel had no previous involvement with the project or knowledge of the children involved. The order of presentation was randomized for each adult, and they were asked to select the best picture to fit in the given slot and to verbalise any observations, such as if they thought 2 or more answers, or none, could be correct. In most cases (551/560) the picture the panel members selected was the one expected by the experimenter according to the originally defined answer scheme.

The study took place in a day school unit for children with impaired communication. All 12 children of the unit were involved, 10 of whom, all boys, were diagnosed either with autism, or behaviours suggestive of autism. We do not claim that these children are representative of all children with autism, but consider them as *individual* cases, from which some generalisations may be made. The remaining 2 children were girls. The children were aged between 5 and 11 years. Twelve visits were made to the unit between February and June 2005.

In order to ground the study in activities relevant to everyday school life, and understand the children's use of TouchStory in the context of their normal behaviours, the children were profiled, involving the children's communication therapist, using a narrative comprehension task based on the work of Paris and Paris (2003.). This involves prompted comprehension questions about a picture story. As children with autism have specific difficulty with 'why', 'what' etc. the questioning strategy was extended to allow the children's therapist to elicit the child's understanding using her usual prompting techniques and the scoring rubric adapted by the experimenter to record both unprompted and prompted answers. The narrative comprehension task was scored by the therapist and the experimenter independently.

The trial using TouchStory consisted of two phases. No adaptation to the individual child took place in the first phase to allow time for TouchStory to become part of the children's established routine, to respond to any initial difficulties, and to create an initial profile of each child. During this phase all children saw the same t-stories at any one visit; new types of t-story were gradually introduced and the actual t-stories shown gradually varied.

The second phase was *adaptive*; the number of t-stories within each category was tailored to each individual child. The purpose of the adaptive phase was that the children would be offered challenging t-stories while retaining the aspect of an enjoyable game. It is central to our approach that we evaluate a simple adaptive formula and increase complexity as necessary. The formula used was, for each t-story type and each child:

- If the child has seen one or zero examples of this type of t-story, or on two or fewer occasions then show two t-stories of this type;
- If the child has had 100% correct answers for this type of t-story on at least two occasions, using a sliding window of 4 occasions, then decrease number of instances of this particular t-story type by 1;
- Otherwise increase the number of instances of this t-story type by 1.

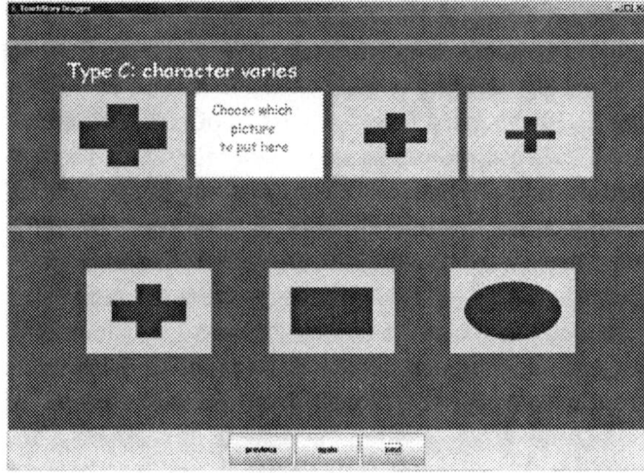

Figure 11.2. The t-story opposite is of type c, which addresses character variability and continuity by presenting a choice among three different characters (in this case different shapes)

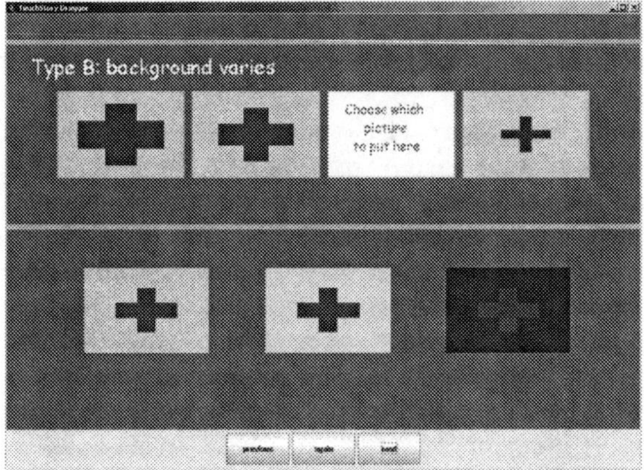

Figure 11.3. Type b addresses background variability and continuity by presenting choice among three different backgrounds (in this case backgrounds of differing colour)

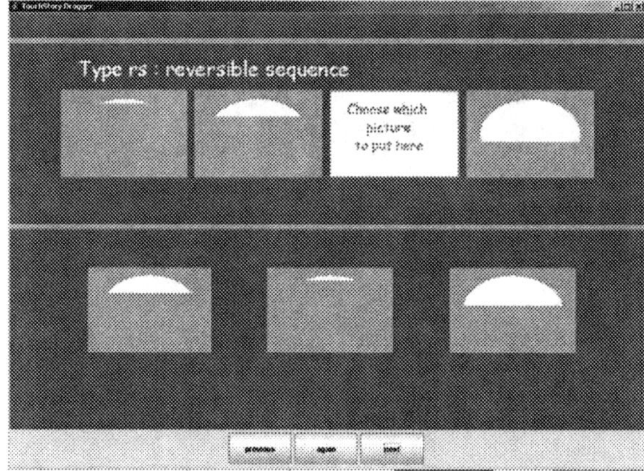

Figure 11.4. The t-story opposite is of type rs, which addresses the sequencing aspect of narrative in a simple form (there is no temporal dimension) by presenting a choice among stages of the sequence

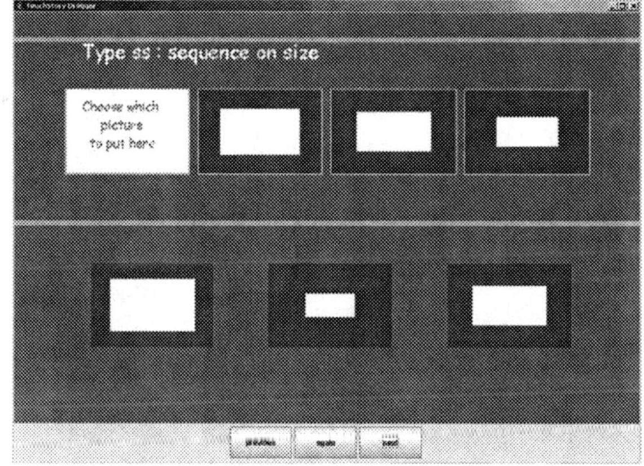

Figure 11.5. The t-story above is of type ss, which is a special form of reversible sequence in which the choice is limited to the size of the character

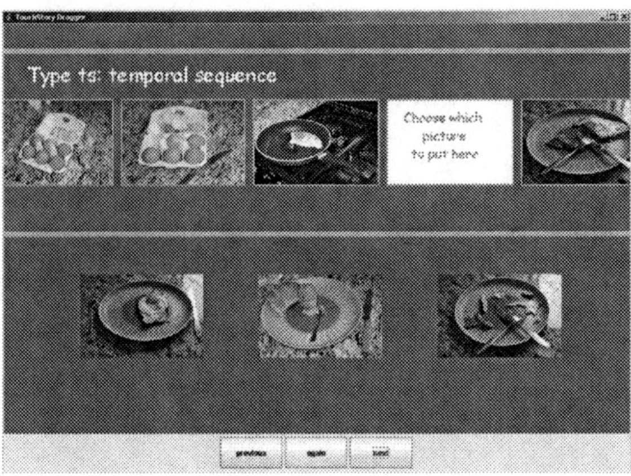

Figure 11.6. The t-story above is of type ts, which addresses temporal aspects sequences of events by presenting a choice among stages of a temporal sequence

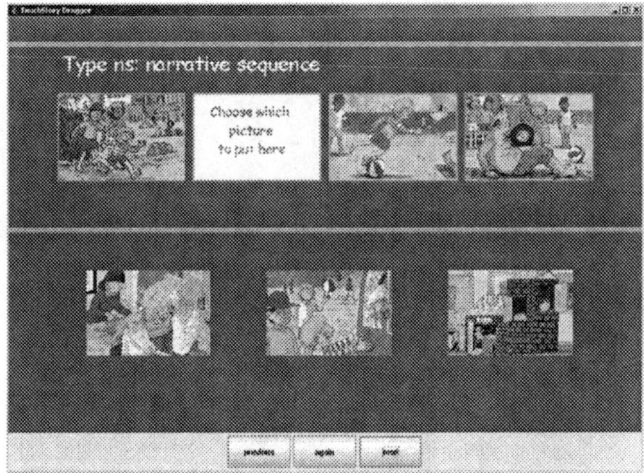

Figure 11.7. The t-story above is of type ns, which are complete mini-narratives extracted from published sources. Illustrations by Alex Brychta from The Hair Cut and The Big Box, by Rod Hunt, illustrated by Alex Brychta (Oxford Reading Tree, 1991), and from The Ice Cream, by Rod Hunt, illustrated by Alex Brychta (Oxford Reading Tree, 2003), copyright © Oxford University Press, reprinted by permission of Oxford University Press.

The profile is then adjusted to fall within the range 12-14 t-stories by generating random numbers to increase or decrease in proportion to the target. Correctness was determined by visual inspection of logs written from the TouchStory programs, (see Table 11.1) which show the child's interaction with TouchStory, in conjunction with notes taken by the experimenter at the time.

The first picture to be docked in the gap was taken as the child's intended answer, this allows the child to touch or move pictures on the workspace as part of the thought process prior to moving one picture into the gap. The adaptive formula was applied by hand between sessions (but will be automated in future work). The order of presentation of t-stories was randomised in the adaptive phase to ameliorate possible effects of fatigue, boredom, early termination of the session, or interference from the mental model engendered by t-stories seen previously in the session.

Table 11.1. TouchStory log for one child attempting one t-story

Log	**Interpretation and comments**
next story eggmeal	t-story 'eggmeal' (shown in Figure 11.2, type ts)
time 11:36:09	is shown at time 11:36:09
option 1 (wrong) selected	the child selects the middle (wrong) option,
option 1 at 433 371	and drags it across the screen,
option 1 at 472 225	through these coordinates
option 1 fitting---------	and docks this, wrong, option in the t-story gap.
option 1 at 482 102	
time 11:36:10	The child realises this is a wrong answer,
option 1 (wrong) selected	and, by choice, drags the option out of the way,
option 1 at 391 172	through these co-ordinates.
option 1 at 329 354	
time 11:36:11	
option 0 (correct) selected	The child now selects option 0, the leftmost one,
option 0 at 356 192	drags it though this coordinate,
option 0 fitting*********	and docks this, correct, option in the t-story gap.

11.5 First Observations

The results showed similarities and differences among the categories and between children, which we illustrate with summary results in Table 11.2. As the adaptive phase means that the number of t-stories shown in each category differs from child to child, the results show the total number of t-stories correct at first attempt as a percentage of the number seen by that child. Consider child ch4, there is a clear distinction between the t-story types he has no difficulty with, and those he does. He finds the narrative sequences difficult, but even more so the temporal sequences; ch1 shows a similar pattern, though gaining higher scores. The profile of ch6 differs, he is relatively successful with narrative sequences, but not with reversible sequences. Children ch2 and ch3 do not have diagnoses of autism. Figure 11.8 shows the effect of the adaptation for each child by showing the percentage of t-stories correct considering all stories up to the numbered visit; thus column *to7* shows the percentage of correct answers up to and including visit 7 *etc.*

Table 11.2. Similarities and differences among the categories and between children: showing for each category, over the whole study, the total number of t-stories correct as a percentage of the number seen by that child

Child	c	b	ss	rs	ts	ns
ch1	100	100	67	72	25	62
ch2	77	67	67	41	36	35
ch3	64	70	75	47	31	30
ch4	100	100	83	54	8	29
ch5	100	100	87	100	100	88
ch6	100	91	100	57	55	71
ch7	No results shown as this child left after visit 5					
ch8	100	78	43	27	67	62
ch9	100	92	78	70	32	48
ch10	100	100	100	73	50	60
ch11	45	50	78	48	60	none seen
ch12	80	64	50	38	0	67

Our expectation was that in the non-adaptive phase we would see a variety of effects, due to the competing effects of increasing familiarity and confidence with TouchStory, and the introduction of new story types. In the adaptive phase we expected an initial decline as the children were exposed to a higher proportion of t-stories they found difficult. In a longer study we would expect to see an eventual upturn if learning took place. The graph shows the expected downturn during the adaptive phase for several children, especially those with a clear and focussed deficit such as children ch1,4,5,8,10. We attibute the upturn for child ch9 to an increased interest in getting the right answer.

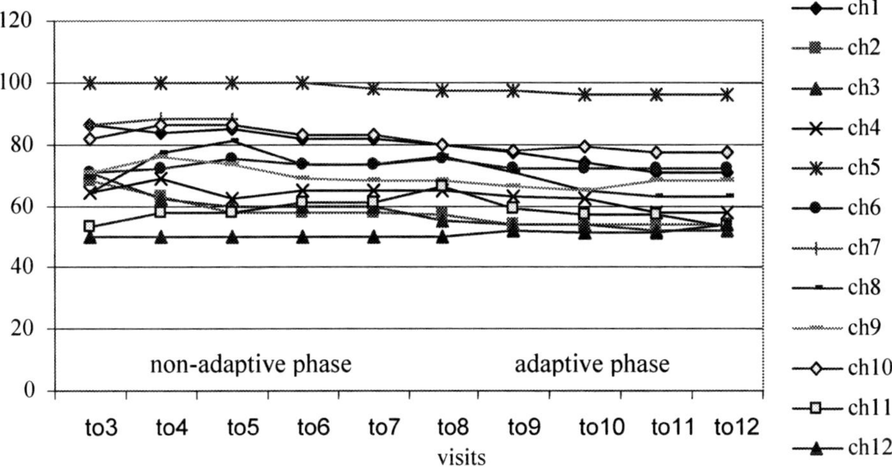

Figure 11.8. Percentage of TouchStory answers correct over all categories for each child as the study progresses

Results relating experiences with TouchStory to real world aspects of narrative comprehension as shown by the adapted Paris and Paris narrative comprehension task (NCT) are as follows. We firstly observe the scores of the two raters of the NCT correlate highly using Spearman rank order correlation r (12) = 0.96, $p<0.05$. The average score given by the two raters was taken as the child's NCT score. The average number of t-stories correctly answered at first attempt, per visit, was taken as a measure of the child's overall success with TouchStory (the TS score). The NCT scores and TS scores were found to correlate significantly at r (12) = 0.82, $p<0.05$. Although this correlation might relate to more general issues of competence and compliance, our results encourage us to think that TouchStory has the potential to illuminate autistic children's understanding of narrative.

11.6 Discussion

For TouchStory to be effective the adaptive formula must be robust. By requiring the child to gain 100% on 2 out of the 4 most recent occasions, we consider that it deals adequately with correct guesses. The results show that it is robust against a child having an 'off-day' and making occasional mistakes. Atypical wrong answers can be seen in the profiles of several children, but because the adaptive formula requires 100% correct answers in 2 of the most recent 4 sessions, they have no effect. It is not robust against a story which the child consistently and atypically gets wrong. This would reduce the outcome to less than 100% every visit it was offered. In future work we will address this. Secondly, the adaptive formula must find a tradeoff between providing rich learning experience for story types that children need to practise, while still presenting sufficient numbers of story types that the children are able to master well, in order to maintain an enjoyable and rewarding context. Last but not least, the learning rate, *i.e.* rate of adaptation during a longitudinal study, could be modified in future work.

11.7 Conclusions and Further Work

The focus of this work is to find ways of enhancing the ability of individual children with autism to deal with narrative. In particular to further understand how to construct computer software that adapts to get the best out of a child in order to directly effect improvement in narrative comprehension or identify aspects of narrative where therapeutic intervention could be applied.

TouchStory is a prototype and we have already touched on a need to further develop *e.g.*, the adaptive formula; but it does seems that TouchStory already goes some way towards identifying aspects of narrative where therapeutic intervention could be applied. However to *directly* effect improvement in narrative comprehension it seems likely that there must be more directed reflection than TouchStory currently provides. Thinking aloud protocols (where users are asked to vocalize their thoughts, feelings, and opinions while interacting with the system), or even informally asking the children questions in the middle of their TouchStory game, is not an option, so more indirect methods of inquiry and pedagogy, possibly including observational analysis will be investigated. Narrative is fundamental to understanding ourselves and the social environment. Interactive computer systems will not be able to provide a quick cure for the narrative deficit found in children in autism. Improvements of children's narrative skills, if any, will only be illuminated in longitudinal studies that also need to show generalisation to other contexts. Thus, the goal is ambitious, but any, even very small steps towards helping children with autism to join in the narrative construction of our (social) world will be an achievement worthwhile, and highlight the challenges of developing computer based interactive learning environments for children with autism.

11.8 Acknowledgements

We thank the staff and pupils of the schools involved. Images from The Haircut, The Ice-cream, and The Big Box (Oxford Reading Tree) are reproduced by permission of the publishers, Oxford University Press.

11.9 References

Abell F, Happe F, Frith U (2000) Do triangles play tricks? Attribution of mental states to animated shapes in normal and abnormal development. Cognitive Development (15): 1–15

Aurora (2000) Available at: http://www.aurora-project.com

Aylett R, Louchart S (2003) Towards a narrative theory of virtual reality. Virtual Reality 7(1): 2–9

Baron-Cohen S (1999) Mindblindness an essay on autism and theory of mind. MIT Press, Cambridge, USA

Bogdashina O (2003) A reconstruction of the sensory world of autism. In: Proceedings of the 7th International Autism-Europe Congress, Portugal

Bruner J (1986) Actual minds, possible worlds. Harvard University Press, Cambridge, USA

Bruner J (1990) Acts of meaning. Harvard University Press, Cambridge, USA

Bruner J (2002) Making stories: law, literature, life. Farrar, Straus and Giro, New York, USA

Bruner J, Feldman C (1993) Theories of mind and the problem of autism. In: Baron-Cohen S *et al.* (eds.) Understanding other minds: perspectives from autism. Oxford University Press, Oxford, UK

Capps L, Losh M, Thurber C (2000) The frog ate the bug and made his mouth sad; narrative competence in children with autism. Journal of Abnormal Child Psychology 18(2): 193–204

Cassell J (2002) Towards a model of technology and literacy development: story listening systems. In: Proceedings of the 2nd Workshop on Narrative and Interactive Learning Environments, Edinburgh, UK

Dautenhahn K (2002) The origins of narrative: in search for the transactional format of narratives in humans and other social animals. International Journal of Cognition and Technology: Co-existence, Convergence, Co-evolution 1(1): 97–123

Davis M, Dautenhahn K, Nehaniv C, Powell S (2004) Towards an interactive system facilitating therapeutic narrative elicitation in autism. In: Proceedings of the 3rd International Conference on Narrative and Interactive Learning Environments, Edinburgh, UK

Frith U (1989) Explaining the enigma. Blackwells Press, Oxford, UK

Graesser AC, Wienner-Hastings K (1999) Situation models and concepts in story comprehension. In: Goldman S *et al.* (eds.) Narrative comprehension, causality and coherence. LEA, Hillsdale, USA

Grandin T (1995) Thinking in pictures. Doubleday, New York, USA

Grynszpan O, Martin J-C, Nadel J (2005) Designing educational software dedicated to people with autism. In: Proceedings of AAATE, Lille, France

Heerera G, Vera L (2005) Abstract concept and imagination teaching through virtual reality in people with autism spectrum disorders. In: Proceedings of AAATE, Lille, France

Hunt R (1991) The hair cut. Illustrations by Alex Brychta. Oxford Reading Tree, Oxford University Press

Hunt R (1991) The big box. Illustrations by Alex Brychta. Oxford Reading Tree, Oxford University Press

Hunt R (2003) The ice cream. Illustrations by Alex Brychta. Oxford Reading Tree, Oxford University Press

Hutto D (2003) Folk psychological narratives and the case of autism. Philosophical Papers 32(3): 345–361

Linde C (1993) Stories, the creation of coherence. Oxford University Press, Oxford, UK

McCloud S (1993) Understanding comics, the invisible art. Harper Perennial, New York, USA

Montemayor J, Druin A, Hendler J (2000) A personal electronic teller of stories. In: Druin A, Hendler J (ed.) Robots for dids – exploring new technologies for learning. Morgan Kaufmann, San Francisco, USA

Moore D, Cheng Y, McGrath P, Powell P (2005) Avatars and sutism. In: Proceedings of AAATE, Lille, France

NAS (2004) National Autistic Society. Available at: http:/www.nas.org.uk

Paris A, Paris SG (2003) Assessing narrative comprehension in young children. Reading Research Quarterly 38(1): 36–76

Porter Abbott H (2002) The Cambridge introduction to narrative. Cambridge University Press, UK

Powell SD (1999) Autism. In: Messer DJ, Millar S (ed.) Developmental psychology. Cambridge University Press, UK

Schank RC (1990) Tell me a story: narrative and intelligence. Northwestern University Press, Evanston, USA

Sehaba K, Courboulay V, Estraillier P (2005) Interactive system by observation and analysis for behaviour for children with autism. In: Proceedings of AAATE, Lille, France

Tager-Flushberg H, Sullivan K (1995) Attributing mental states to story characters: a comparison of narratives produced by autistic and mentally retarded individuals. Applied Psycholinguistics 16: 241–256

Wing L (1996) The autistic spectrum: a guide for parents and professionals. Constable, London, UK

Part III

Assistive Technology and Rehabilitation Robotics

Chapter 12

Collaborative Visual-servoing of the MANUS Manipulator

F. Liefhebber, B.J.F. Driessen and A.H.C. Thean

12.1 Introduction

The rehabilitation robot Manus (Verburg, 1996) is an assistive device for severely motor handicapped users. With it, users can perform daily tasks that would otherwise be impossible or would require the help of other persons. Manus has eight degrees of freedom (DOFs); three for positioning the gripper, three for rotating the gripper about three axes, one for opening the gripper and one external lift.

Because of its eight DOFs, Manus is a complex device, which is sometimes cumbersome to control for persons with very limited residual functionality. A challenge for the research community is to develop assisting technology for controlling complex devices like Manus in an intuitive way. Here, a method is proposed, which uses sensors (such as cameras, force torque sensors, and infrared distance sensors) to ease the control of the system. Manus must operate in a challenging unstructured environment and it is not our goal to make it fully autonomous. Our philosophy is that the user actively controls the device and retains supervision in all circumstances. The combination of direct user control and autonomous sensor control is known in literature as "collaborative control".

This paper is organised as follows. The next paragraph describes the general architecture of the proposed controller. Next, a vision-based controller, which is the central part of the collaborative controller, is discussed in detail. Finally, the user interface is described followed by a description of the first user trials.

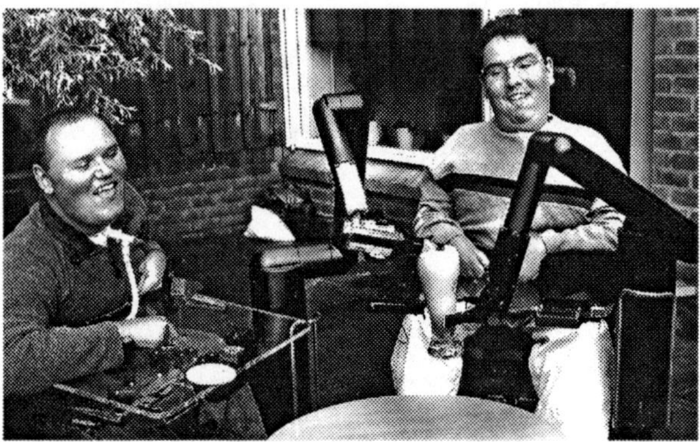

Figure 12.1. Two Manus end-users

12.2 Collaborative Control

The main difference between a collaborative control system and a standard fully autonomous control system is that collaborative control requires a higher degree of involvement from the user in the control loop. The role of the user is not limited to issuing prescribed high-level commands. Instead, the user actively takes part in controlling the robot. Figure 12.2 shows the general architecture of our collaborative controller. The manipulator (Manus) has to interact with objects that exist in the environment (a cup on a table, a book on a shelf, a spoon in a cutlery tray, *etc.*). The user can see both the manipulator and the objects in the environment. Based on his/her observations he/she can issue commands to the manipulator through a user interface. Sensors are used for measuring different aspects of the manipulator or the environment. Examples are angle encoders that determine the pose of the robot, a force-torque sensor that measures the interaction force between object and robot, or a camera, which measures the pose of an object with respect to the camera. Note that sensors can be integrated in the manipulator as well as in the environment. The sensor outputs are fused in the sensor fusion block to obtain a more reliable representation of the world. The output of the sensor fusion block is fed to the control fusion block, which controls Manus.

The sensor fusion block applies Kalman filtering to the measurement of the camera and the distance sensor, which results in a more reliable estimation of the current state (*e.g.* pose of the object with respect to the manipulator) of the system. This block can also be used to fuse multiple cameras each with a different position and direction and select the best view of the environment. The outputs of the sensor fusion (Ng, 2003) block are various state variables, which each require a different type of controller. The control fusion block contains these controllers and combines their outputs to a consistent control input to the Manus. The fusion of the various control laws (controllers) takes care of two issues: distribution of the DOFs between the control laws and minimisation of the coupling between the control laws. For example, a camera is used to control the roll, pitch and yaw, a distance sensor is used to control the Z position and the user controls the X and Y position.

The next section describes in detail how this architecture is implemented in the Manus control system and includes a description of the user interface. Particular attention is paid to vision based control.

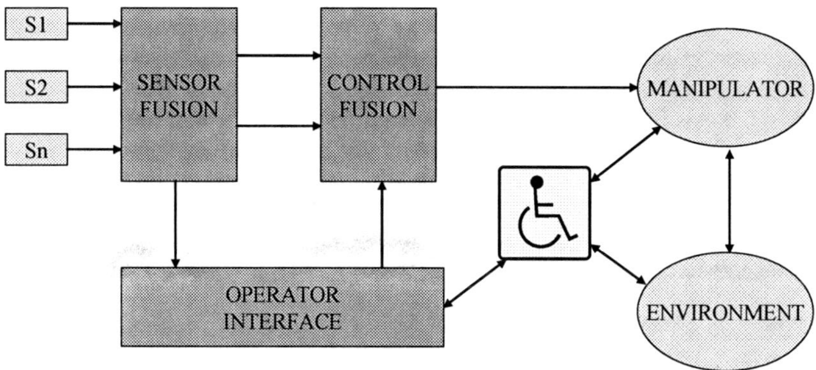

Figure 12.2. Collaborative control scheme

12.3 Vision Based Control

12.3.1 Visual Servoing

The term "visual-servoing" (Corke, 1996) is a description of all control-strategies which use visual information for controlling the position and orientation of a manipulator. Two main approaches can be identified: position-based visual servoing (PBVS) and image-based visual servoing (IBVS). In PBVS (Malis, 2002), the 3D position and orientation (pose) of an object is estimated using image features and this estimate is used for control. In IBVS (Espiau *et al.*, 1992; Hashimoto, 1999; Malis, 2002), the image features themselves are used for the control in order to position the robot. Image features such as colour, texture and interest points (*e.g.* corners) can be used.

Many approaches to visual servoing rely heavily on *a priori* knowledge. For example model-based PBVS (Malis, 2002) requires a 3D model of the object of interest and model-free PBVS (Chaumette and Malis, 2000) and general IBVS (Malis, 2002) require a teach-and-learn procedure in advance. During a teach-and-learn phase, the desired image (or desired values) and templates are learnt from the object. This learnt data is put in a database which will hold the required data for all objects. For our application the controller has to operate in an unstructured environment, with a high number of objects, some of which will only ever be manipulated once (*e.g.* dining in a restaurant). This makes the use of *a priori* knowledge problematic and therefore we have designed a vision-based-control technique which does not require any *a priori* knowledge.

Visual servoing on the basis of image moments (Chaumette, 2002) does not require much *a priori* knowledge because the desired features are the same for all objects and no templates of the objects are required. In the field of computer vision, image-moments are commonly used to describe the position, size, shape and orientation of objects in an image. Image-moments can be calculated from a binary 2D area, which represents the object of interest in an image. The segmentation of the object of interest from the captured image is done on basis of the same colour (hue and saturation) and intensity (value) in the HSV colourspace.

In an extensive modelling of moments (m_{ij}) and central-moments (μ_{ij}) is described (Chaumette, 2002). The indices i and j of m_{ij} and μ_{ij} represent the order in the x and y direction respectively. In our case we use combinations of image moments, which contain information about the position of the object with respect to the camera. The computer vision system calculates the centre-of mass s_x (= m_{10} / m_{00}) and s_y (= m_{01} / m_{00}), surface s_a (= m_{00}) and s_ϕ, which is defined as:

$$s_\phi = \frac{1}{2}\arctan\left(\frac{2\mu_{11}}{-|\mu_{20}-\mu_{02}|}\right). \tag{1}$$

The visual-servoing controller aims to bring the features $\mathbf{s} = [\, s_x, s_y, s_a, s_\phi]^T$ to their desired value $\mathbf{s}^*$ by controlling the position and orientation of the manipulator. We would like to position the object in the centre of the camera at a certain distance with vertical orientation (necessary to grasp the object with a parallel gripper); this pose results in the desired values $\mathbf{s}^*$ of $[0, 0, a^*, 0]^T$. The desired surface a^* and current distance to the object are estimated by a depth-from-motion algorithm based on an extended Kalman filter (Ng, 2003).

Linear visual-servoing control laws, such as PID (Proportional, Integration and Differential control) or state-feedback, will result in poor closed-loop performance or instability, because of the non-linear perspective camera mapping. This mapping, from camera velocity to features, can easily be described by the so-called image Jacobian (**L**), which fulfils the following equation:

$$\dot{\mathbf{s}} = \mathbf{L}\mathbf{v}_{cam} \tag{2}$$

where $\dot{\mathbf{s}}$ is the time variation of the features, **L** is the image Jacobian and $\mathbf{v}_{cam}$ is the velocity screw of the camera. This image Jacobian depends on the distance from the camera to the object and the current feature values. Mathematical modelling of the image Jacobian is described in Espiau *et al.* (1992), Hashimoto (1999) and Chaumette (2002).

The pseudo-inverse ($^+$) of the image Jacobian can be used in a control law to compensate for the perspective mapping of the camera and the cross coupling between the DOFs and the features. We use the following IBVS control law:

$$\mathbf{v}_{cam} = -\lambda\mathbf{L}^+\left(\mathbf{s}^* - \mathbf{s}\right). \tag{3}$$

which results in asymptotically stable behaviour and the cross coupling between the features is minimal (Chaumette, 2002). This IBVS control law will try to minimise the error between the measured and desired features and it will result in a trajectory in the image space which is as short as possible (Chaumette, 1995).

Which DOFs are controlled can be specified by a selection-matrix (**M**) so that the control law becomes:

$$\mathbf{v}_{cam} = -\lambda(\mathbf{LM})^{+}\left(\mathbf{s}^{*} - \mathbf{s}\right). \tag{4}$$

In case more DOFs are controlled than the number of features that are used (rank(**LM**) > dim(**s**)), the columns of the matrix (**LM**) are dependent. This dependency can be exploited to fulfil constraints or to perform a secondary control task (Marchand and Hager, 1998). In our case, a secondary control law is used to fix the orientation of the manipulator on the basis of the known kinematics of the arm. The control space (span) of the secondary control law should be perpendicular to the control space of the visual-servoing control law in order to guarantee that these two control laws will not conflict with each other. The secondary control law will have the following form:

$$\mathbf{v}_2 = \lambda_2\left(\mathbf{M} - (\mathbf{LM})^{+}\mathbf{L}\right)\mathbf{e}_2 \tag{5}$$

The combination of the visual-servoing-controller and the secondary controller is able to control all DOFs simultaneously (see Figure 12.3). The number of DOFs that are controlled simultaneously depend on the distance to the target. The trajectory of the end-effector can be influenced, during the approach of an object, by this distance dependant assignment of the DOFs to each controller.

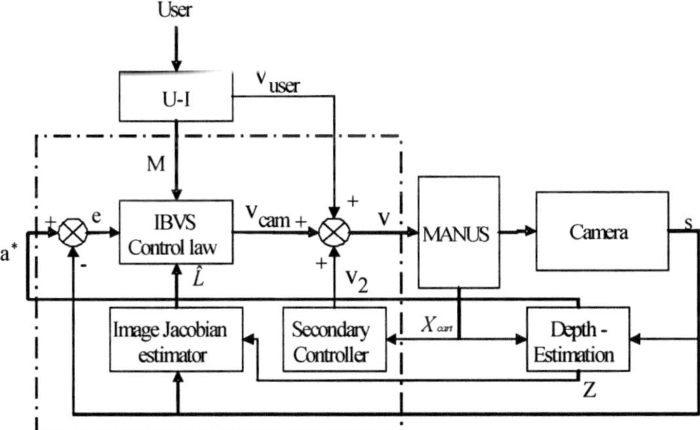

Figure 12.3. Implementation of the collaborative controller, consisting of an IBVS-controller, secondary kinematics controller, depth estimator and user input

12.3.2 Camera Set-up

The camera configuration and exact placement of the camera in the system have consequences for the functionality and behaviour of vision-based control. Therefore several camera set-ups have been investigated. To avoid occlusions of the camera by the arm an eye-in-hand camera-configuration (camera is attached to the gripper) was chosen instead of a stand-alone configuration (camera has a fixed position). For the eye-in-hand configuration three locations (see Figure 12.4a) of camera on the gripper are interesting.

The classification of the 'best' eye-in-hand camera location is difficult, because it requires a choice between desired behaviour of the IBVS-controller and the ability to use the camera. For location a, the fingers of the gripper block the field of view of the camera more than is the case for location b. The task of an IBVS-controller is described in the image space and doesn't have any knowledge about the Cartesian 3D space. This can cause unnecessary long and strange trajectories in the Cartesian space. For IBVS, the location of the camera is optimal in the centre of the gripper (location a or b). In this way it is straightforward to drive the gripper towards the centre of the object. Also, for objects at large distances, the gripper approaches the object in an intuitive way (*i.e.* straight line directed towards the object). The disadvantage of location a and b, is that once an object has been grasped, the field of view of the camera will be blocked totally by the object.

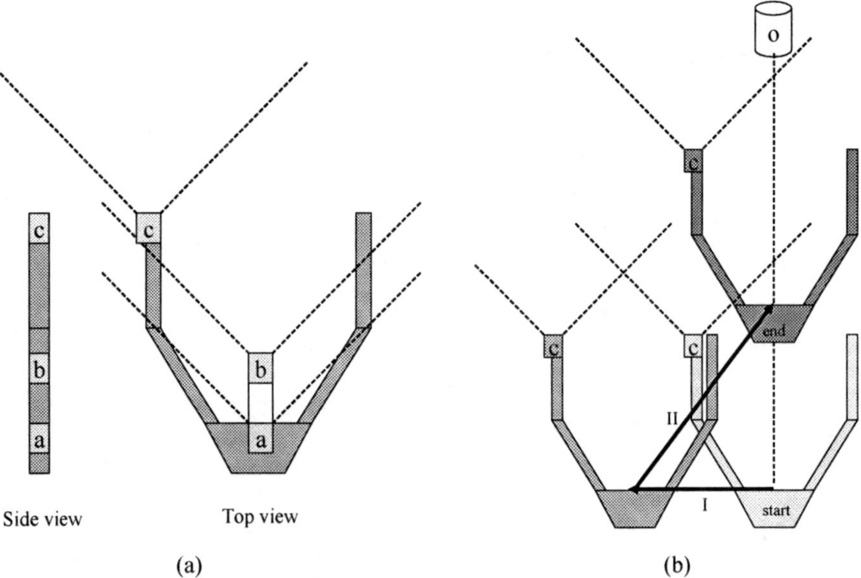

Figure 12.4. (a) Camera locations for the eye-in-hand configuration. (b) Undesired behaviour if the visual servo drives the centre of the object to an offset position in the image plane. After the visual servo is activated, trajectory I will be performed and during the approach to the object, it will follow trajectory II.

In the case where the camera is placed in the finger instead of the gripper (location a and b), the visual servoing algorithm drives the *finger* (rather than the centre of the gripper) towards the object. For actually grasping an object, the user must first move the gripper sideways, after which the final approach can be accomplished. This extra motion is undesired, since it requires extra user input. Driving the centre of the object not to the centre of the image plane, but to a small offset position on the image plane will eventually place the gripper in front of the object. However, at large distances, counter-intuitive motions will occur, since the servo immediately tries to position the centre of the object at the predefined position in the image plane (see Figure 12.4b). This behaviour can be avoided if the distance towards the object is known. The required feature position (Mezouar and Chaumette, 2002) can be defined as a function of the object distance.

For Manus, the ability to use the camera as sensor for vision-based control or as an aid to the user once an object is grasped is of most importance. Therefore, location c was chosen as the final camera location.

12.4 User Interfacing

For controlling the user interface, the wheelchair joystick is used, supplemented by an extra switch. In this user interface (Tijsma *et al.*, 2005) three control modes are implemented:

- Cartesian control mode with respect to world coordinates;
- Cartesian control with respect to the task frame, referred to as 'Pilot mode'
- Joint mode, in which all the joints of the MANUS can be controlled.

The object selection procedure of the computer vision is activated when the user presses the switch. The location of the object of interest can be pinpointed on the user's screen, using the joystick. Pressing the switch again, the computer vision will start with the segmentation of the pinpointed object and gives feedback to the user by highlighting the segmented area (the object) in the image. Meanwhile the vision-based-controller is activated and will move the gripper to the desired position with respect to the pinpointed object. The controller can be deactivated at any time by pressing the switch again. The number of DOFs that are controlled by the visual servoing controller can be adjusted in accordance with the wishes of the user. The graphical user interface (displayed in Figure 12.5) is displayed on a 7-inch widescreen TFT display. In the textboxes the control modes are displayed. The active control mode is highlighted in pale grey. All the other menus are displayed in dark grey.

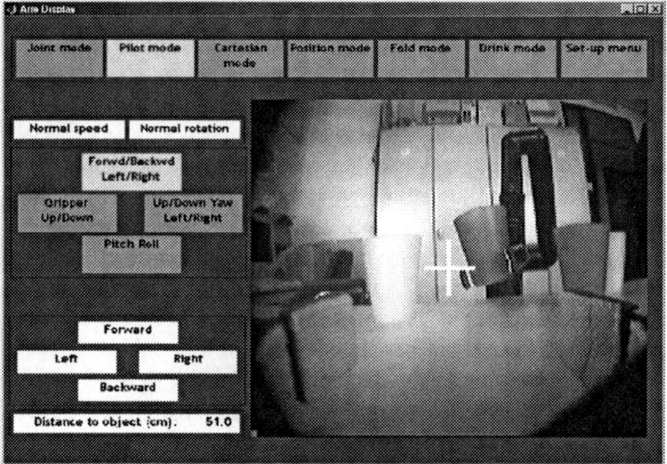

Figure 12.5. Visual servoing user interface

The control modes that can be selected are aligned in a row. This row is displayed in the upper part of the figure. Giving a fast flick with the joystick to the left or to the right allows the user to scroll through these control modes. Giving a fast flick downwards can activate a control mode. If the control mode is active, the sub modes of this control mode will be displayed to the left of the camera image of the gripper-mounted camera. The user can change from one mode to the other by giving a fast flick in the direction of the desired control mode as displayed in the figure.

12.5 Evaluations

The total system was evaluated by four end-users (Tijsma *et al.*, 2005). All users were experienced Manus users, but none had experience of using Manus with the current camera and visual servoing system. To allow the users to get familiar with the camera system, at first no visual servoing functionality was offered. Using the camera image users were able to pick up objects which could not be directly seen by them. However, guiding the manipulator to the required position was far from straightforward if only the camera information was used as user-feedback signal. The main user problems were:

- The users were not used to controlling the manipulator in "Pilot-mode" (controlling the manipulator with respect to the tool-camera frame).
- The users found it difficult to relate the camera view to the motion of the manipulator.

More training by users will reduce the cognitive load, but this task will remain difficult.

During successive trials the visual servoing functionality was offered. The task for the user was to pick up various objects from a difficult starting position. The main goal of these experiments was to investigate the usability of the vision-based-controller in combination with simultaneous user input

The user was able to complete the evaluation tasks successfully with the collaborative controller. The required time to approach the object was drastically reduced, but the required time to select the object in camera view almost cancelled out this task time improvement. For each task, a technical assistant had to manually set up the distribution of manual DOFs (XYZ or YPR) and automatic DOFs (YPR or XYZ). It was found that using visual servoing, the cognitive load (Tijsma *et al.*, 2005) required for picking up the cup was reduced significantly. All users, who were relatively sceptical at the start of the experiments, reacted positively to the new development. However, it was clear that the robustness of the vision system needs to be improved in order to make it more versatile.

During the evaluation, the users appreciated the new graphical user interface and stated that the layout of the interface was very clear. The size of the camera-view is a little bit too small and therefore it is sometimes hard to see the object of interest. To increase the size of the camera-view, but not the size of the tft-display, we will use the entire display for the camera-view and overlay it with transparent buttons and textboxes.

12.6 Conclusions and Future Research

A system is presented which applies the collaborative control paradigm on the MANUS system. The collaborative controller uses the image-based visual servoing approach based on image moments. A nice and required property of these features is that the desired values are the same for all types of object and therefore it can operate in unknown and unstructured environments. Since the number of controllable DOFs is higher than the number of image features used by the visual servoing algorithm, a secondary controller can constrain the position of some DOFs in desired positions (*e.g.* gripper vertical).

The Manus is equipped with an eye-in-hand camera which was located in the centre of the wrist. A disadvantage of this camera location is that the camera is blocked when an object is grasped. The location of the camera in the fingertips will not have this disadvantage, but it can result in counter-intuitive motions of the vision-based controller. The tracking of object features is carried out using colour segmentation and some moments-based properties are calculated on the basis of the segmented area.

To increase the robustness of the system more research is required on the computer vision area. To improve the performance and robustness of the computer vision, we will investigate the fusion of multiple cameras (eye-in-hand and stand-alone) and the use of different algorithms, which can better track textured objects.

The resulting behaviour and functionality of a camera in the fingertip (and in combination with another camera) requires more research and the integration of this camera in the finger of the Manus gripper will also be a challenge.

In the near future more evaluations with users will be used to test the functionality and usability of this collaborative system and to improve the user interface.

12.7 References

Chaumette F (1997) Potential problems of stability and convergence in image-based and position-based visual servoing. In: Proceedings of the Workshop on Vision and Control, Block Island, USA

Chaumette F, Malis E (2000) 2½ D visual servoing: a possible solution to improve image-based and position-based visual servoings. In: Proceedings of the 2000 IEEE International Conference on Robotics and Automation, San Francisco, USA

Chaumette F (2002) A first step towards visual servoing using image moments. In: Proceedings of the 2002 IEEE/ RSJ International Conference on Intelligent Robots and Systems, EPFL, Switzerland

Corke PI (1996) Visual control of robots: 'high-performance visual servoing'. Research Studies Press LTD., Taunton, UK

Driessen B, Liefhebber F, ten Kate T, van Woerden J (2005) Collaborative control of the Manus. In: Proceedings of ICORR 2005, Chicago, USA

Espiau B, Chaumette F, Rives P (1992) A new approach to visual servoing in robotics. IEEE Transactions on Robotics and Automation 8(3): 313–326

Hashimoto K (1999) Observer-based visual servoing. In: Ghosh BK *et al.* (eds.) Control in robotics and automation. Academic Press, London, UK

Malis E (2002) Survey of vision-based robot control. Available at: http://www.isa.umh.es/temas/vs/doc/Ezio%20Malis%20Survey.pdf

Marchand E, Hager GD (1998) Dynamic sensor planning in visual servoing. In: Proceedings of the IEEE International Conference on Robotics and Automation, Leuven, Belgium

Marchand E, Chaumette F (2004) Features tracking for visual servoing purposes. In: Kragic D, Christensen H (eds.) Advances in robot vision – from domestic environments to medical applications. Sendai, Japan

Mezouar Y, Chaumette F (2002) Path planning for robust image-based-visual-servoing. IEEE Transactions on Robotics and Automation 18(4): 534–549

Ng GW (2003) Intelligent systems – fusion, tracking and control. Research Studies Press Ltd., Taunton, UK

Tijsma HA, Liefhebber F, Versluis AHG, Herder JL (2005) Evaluation of new user interface features for the Manus robot arm. In: Proceedings of ICORR 2005, Chicago, USA

Tijsma HA, Liefhebber F, Versluis AHG, Herder JL (2005) A framework of interface improvements for designing new user interfaces for the Manus robot arm. In: Proceedings of ICORR 2005, Chicago, USA

Verburg G, Kwee H, Wisanaka A, Cheetham A, van Woerden J (1996) MANUS: the evolution of an assistive technology. Technology and Disability 5(2): 217–228

Chapter 13

User-centred Approach to the Design and Evaluation of a Stair-climbing Aid

R.E. Mayagoitia, S. Kitchen, J. Harding, R. King and A. Turner-Smith

13.1 Introduction

In a precursor to this paper, done under the EQUAL programme of the EPSRC and published in 2002, a focus group methodology was used for older people to identify and describe the nature of the mobility-related problems that they encounter, and to then put forward ideas for their resolution, which might usefully be addressed by innovative assistive technology research. The three main problems identified using thematic analysis were: bending and reaching, stair climbing and getting information (Seale *et al.*, 2002). The development of a stair-climbing device was taken up in a second phase of that project.

A simple wooden prototype was made and the participants of the focus groups were invited to trials where their feedback was collected individually using a five-minute semi-structured interview. The thematic analysis of the comments revealed that the group members responded favourably to the principle of the stair-climbing aid, and came up with a number of suggestions for improvements (McCreadie *et al.*, 2002). These were taken up and a new project to further develop the stair-climbing device was proposed and funded under the Health Technologies Development Programme of the Department of Health. The project partners were Stannah Stairlifts, Harding Industrial Design, Hammersmith and Fulham Disability Adaptations Unit and King's College London. Herein is reported the user-centred approach to this third phase of development.

The rationale for continuing with the development of a stair-climbing device includes considerations such as the following. The Department of Trade and Industry (DTI, 2003) found that in the United Kingdom approximately 20 000 hospitalisations and 900 deaths occur each year in those aged 65 and over due to falls on stairs or steps. It has been shown by Shimada *et al.* (2003) that exercise, such as stair climbing, can improve the general balance of an older person and therefore reduces the likelihood of a fall. Hill *et al.* (2000) agreed with this and also suggested that 'There may also be a psychological effect accompanying reduced stair use, leading to increased apprehension on the occasions on which they are used'.

The new, purely mechanical, counter-balanced, ratchet mechanism device (Figure 13.1) was designed to help frail elderly people climb stairs more safely whilst still maintaining the benefits of stair climbing as a form of exercise. The device folds away when not in use. To ascend, the user simply pushes on the bar for support while taking ascending steps using a swing to stairs climbing strategy. To descend, the user rocks the bar to disengage the stop, pushes down until the next stop and then takes a step down, also using a swing to movement. The user is enveloped by the bar, which besides providing upper limb support can also catch a user, if he or she trips or slips on the stairs. A number of similar devices (The Stair Bar at http://www.stairbar.co.uk/) exist but none as yet have become commercially successful. The aim of the part of the project presented here was to elicit and examine the opinions of older subjects of a prototype assistive device designed to provide support during active ascent and descent of stairs.

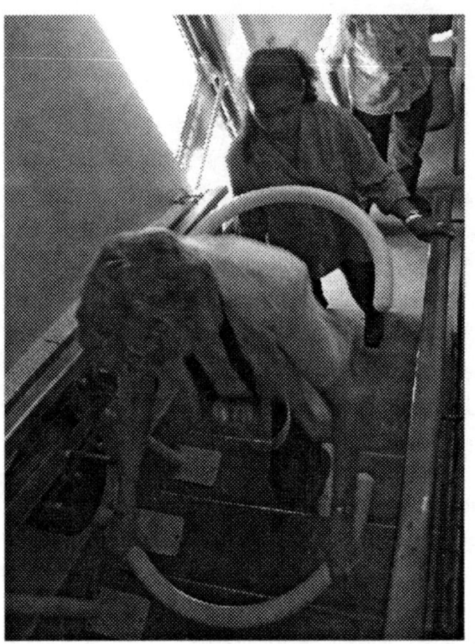

A. Ascent

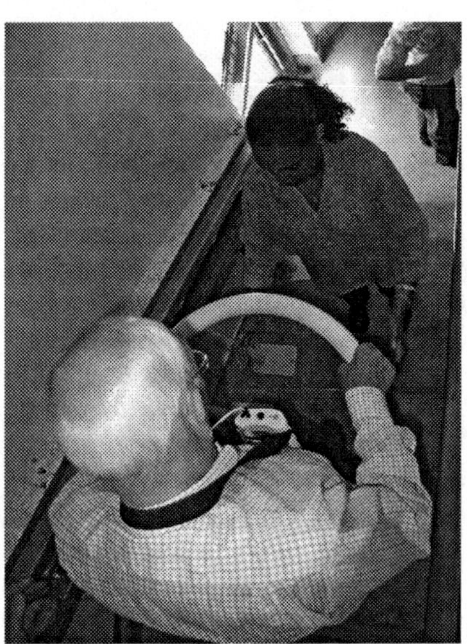

B. Descent

Figure 13.1. Photographs of volunteers using the stair-climbing device (Patent King's College London)

13.2 Methods

The project received approval number 04/05-08 from King's College London Research Ethics Committee. All the participants had the full testing procedure explained to them, had their questions answered (if any) and were provided with an information sheet. Written consent was obtained prior to commencement. The volunteers also signed a non-disclosure agreement regarding the design of the device they were testing.

There were three sources of data during a testing session: clinical tests, biomechanical tests and interview, conducted in that order. The clinical tests were randomised and consisted of Berg balance scale, timed up and go, six minute walk (Steffen *et al.*, 2002), and the SF-36™ health questionnaire (Quality Metric Incorporated). Care was taken that volunteers had enough time to rest before proceeding to the next stage. Bio-mechanical tests consisted of stair climbing a flight of steps without and with the support of the new device while wearing a traixial accelerometer and gyroscope sensor (XSens MT9, Xsens BV) at the small of the back. The semi-structured interviews were carried out after the use of the device.

This present study used a concrete staircase, consisting of eight steps, with handrails on either side, diagrammed in Figure 13.2. The staircase was located in a sheltered accommodation building where several of the volunteers lived.

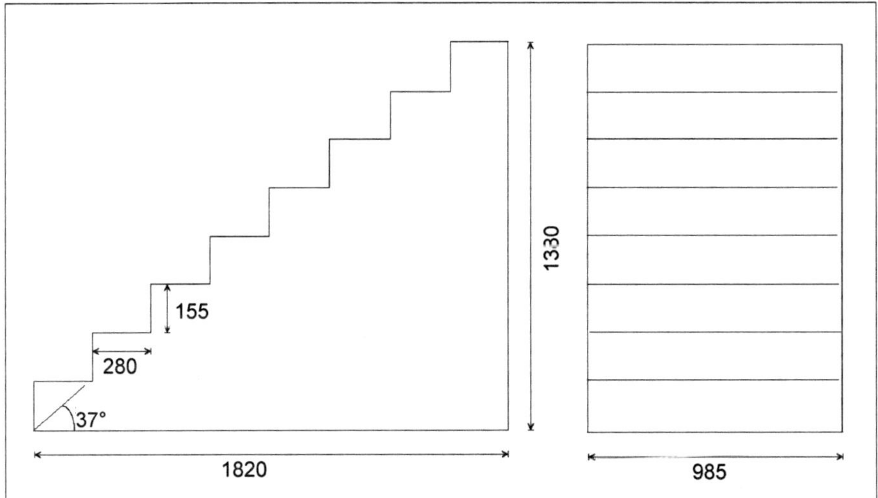

Figure 13.2. Diagram of stairs: all dimensions are in mm

Semi-structured interviews were used to elicit the opinions of subjects who had tested or viewed the stairclimbing device. Following a further explanation of the purpose of this element of the study, consent to take notes was obtained immediately before the interviews. Each interview took approximately 10-15 minutes.

Key probe topics included: What are your first impressions of the new device? What do you think about the way it looks? Is it suitable for your home? Was the device easy/difficult to use? (Entry/exit, turning, stops, bar, ascent/descent.) Did you feel safe/confident using the device?

13.3 Subjects

Twenty-six of a total of 28 participants in the study agreed to be interviewed about their views of the stair-climbing device. They were aged between 62 and 94 years; 15 were female; all were living in the community or in sheltered housing, without obvious cognitive impairment; some required the use of either handrails or other assistive device, such as a stick, to ascend and descend stairs. All subjects were occupying single storey accommodation. Nine subjects noted that they had had difficulty with stairs prior to moving to their present home, while seven reported no such problems. The remainder did not comment on this area. Six reported no concurrent medical conditions; seven reported one and the remainder multiple health problems. Five subjects reported spinal, arthritic, heart or "on the day" problems (*e.g.* "I don't feel good today".) Three were diabetic and three had self-confessed balance difficulties. Other conditions included stroke, polio, hip replacement, polymyalgia or old fractures. Five reported using a stick for walking and one a rolator.

Two subjects declined to use the device (subjects 7 and 10) but agreed to be interviewed; 24 were able to use the stair climber to both ascend and descend the single flight of eight stairs.

13.4 Analysis

Open answers were derived and content analysis used to examine the material. Responses were read and emerging themes noted and defined. The data was then coded according to these themes. The themes, the definitions and the coded material were then given to two independent assessors to check for validity of interpretation. Full agreement between assessors was obtained after discussion.

13.5 Results

Ten categories were identified from the results; in addition, a number of general remarks were made. Numbers of subjects are indicated by (n=); statements by (s=). Individual statements are coded by subject, then statement number, *e.g.* 2.1.

First impressions: subjects were asked for their first impression of the device. Twenty-eight statements were made by 22 subjects. *E.g.*twenty statements were positive and indicated that the subject found the device useful. Examples include:

"Very good device for people with difficulties up and down stairs" (2.1) "Very good … excellent … something new" (8.2) "I got on quite well with the device …" (15.1). Three statements expressed some reservations, one from a volunteer who did not test the device. For example: "My first impression was that it looked awful. I would hate to have it in my own home because friends would say I was getting old and decrepit". Other statements indicated that the device would be useful or that they would use it (s=3), was less clumsy than a chair-lift (s=3) and one subject suggested that it would be cheaper.

Appearance: 12 statements were made by nine subjects about the appearance of the stair-climbing device. Three subjects suggested that it was rather big, one that it was clumsy and one that it would depend on the home situation: 'if you had two flights of stairs'' (19.6). Two subjects indicated that appearance was not important while two others made explicitly positive comments: "aesthetics are fine" (6.19) and "I liked the bar … it has a nice sort of curve to it" (17.3).

Suitability for home use: 20 statements were made by 16 subjects about this area. Fifteen of the responses suggested that the device would be used if there was a need or indicated reasons why it might be successful. For example: "I'd have it in my home … be independent …" (6.16) "the housing I am moving to has a very narrow staircase so it might be better than a stair-lift" (17.10). One noted that it would only be used as an interim device. The four remaining statements related to size. Three were value neutral but suggested that it might be too big, would need a large staircase or would pose a problem if the bar "needed holding up". The remaining subject stated that they would not use the device in their home because it was too big.

Noise: 13 subjects made 14 statements about the level of noise produced in use. Ten noted that the device was noisy or very noisy. Ten indicated that the noise occurring was not a major problem, though one noted that "you cannot hear yourself think" (17.4) when moving at speed. One noted that she did not "even think of it" (5.8).

Difficult / easy to use: 12 subjects made 25 statements about this area. Thirteen statements noted that the device was easy or simple to use – "fairly simple (6.11)", "easy to push up and down with one hand" (8.12) and "easy to get in and out of" (15.4). This last subject also indicated that it was "big and hard to push". Six statements indicated some difficulty; for example, "heavy to push" (2.2) and "a bit complicated to start with" (11.4).

Entry, exit and turning: 16 subjects made 23 statements. All statements were positive, indicating plenty of space to enter and leave the device and adequate room for turning at the top of the stairs. Examples include: "I got in and out without difficulty" (13.5) "Enough room to turn around at the top ... not restricted by the aid (5.10)"

Ascent and descent: 14 subjects made 19 statements. Generally this was considered to be satisfactory, though 8 subjects explicitly noted that coming down was more difficult than going up. Reasons for this included concern "coming down may be a worry" (6.14)), having to lean forward (15.7) and "maybe the steps were not in the right position" (16.5). Three found both directions equally easy while one found ascent difficult. This subject noted that they did not benefit from the device greatly on ascent – "I felt going up I tended to be pulling the equipment up rather than pushing it and felt I didn't pull it as far forward as needed so didn't benefit from leaning on the device" (1.5)

Stops: 11 subjects each made single statements all indicating that the stops were satisfactory. They were reported to be safe, in the right position and firm and secure. One subject noted the need to learn how to use them (12.8).

Bar (shape, weight, position): this was an area of interest to the subjects with 20 making 47 statements, the majority of which indicated that the bar was well positioned, the diameter of the bar and grip good and the shape satisfactory. Twelve statements referred to the grip as good, firm, solid or strong. Seven subjects noted that the bar was the right size, two considered it too large and one too small. The height of the bar (7 respondents) and distance from the user (5 respondents) were considered satisfactory; 1 subject found the height too low (12.6), another that it would be good to be able to adjust this dimension and one the length too great. The one problem identified was the perceived weight of the bar – though it was not always clear if this was actually the weight or the force need to push the bar. Four subjects noted this – "the bar was a bit heavy (9.3)". Two further subjects noted it was hard to push. Two specifically noted that it was not heavy. All remaining statements were positive or neutral in their content, noting that they could position it as they wished (n=2), it would fit different people (n=1) – though it might need to be larger 'for Hattie Jaques' (n=1), and it was "about right" or "just right" (n=2). One noted that the cradle effect was good.

Safe / confident / in control: 21 subjects made 33 statements, and of these 17 indicated that the device was perceived as safe and secure. Two further subjects noted that they felt in good control of the device. Two statements suggested the subjects did not feel this way: "Not very confident" (8.17) "I did feel it might run away with me" (14.14). One subject asked questions about safety and two noted that it was essential.

General remarks: 35 general remarks were made by 17 subjects. General, positive remarks accounted for 16 statements. Subjects noted that the device allowed them to continue to "use their legs" (n= 3) and was not as cumbersome as a chair lift (n= 3), though one noted that with a stair-lift (chair version) all you had to do was "just sit in it and press a button" (19.7)). Two subjects noted that the device tested was a prototype and that they therefore expected slight changes to be made; one suggested "plastic for lightness and sound" (6.21) and another that the device should be "lighter and smaller" (15.12). Three others indicated that they could not think of any ways to improve it. One subject each reported that it slowed down the speaker, might be better for younger people who were less easily confused, or particularly useful on steep steps.

In contrast with the user's perspective, a report from the occupational therapy partners at Hammersmith and Fulham concluded that, "as the prototype was refined, it became apparent to us that our initial safety concerns had been addressed ... and the final prototype appeared to be a useful aid for stair climbing." They summarised their point of view in Table 13.1.

Table 13.1. Summary of pros and cons by occupational therapy partners

Pros	Cons
Non electrical - no ongoing running costs for the user	Specialist required to install and remove product
Should be relatively easy to install and remove and can be re-cycled. Therefore more cost effective for Local Government	Only for a straight staircase
	Fairly 'person specific' in terms of height settings
Maintains stair climbing ability	Stair rail has to be removed
Safer for a carer when guiding a person up and down stairs	Unsuitable for narrow staircases
User controls the speed of ascent and decent	Requires a level of cognitive ability to be used safely
Potential for use in a rehab environment as well	

13.6 Discussion

The prototype was perceived to be easy to use, though some technical problems arose during the tests which made a number of runs increasingly stiff or 'heavy'. This issue would have to be addressed in the next prototype, as most subjects who might use the device are likely to be fragile or disabled in some way. However, most subjects seemed to see beyond this immediate problem in their response to the device.

One of the benefits of the device is that it allows the subject to remain actively climbing stairs, a factor that can contribute to the maintenance of fitness in an older person. A number of subjects noted this as a benefit. A small number of subjects suggested populations that might benefit from the help offered; these included the fragile, anybody requiring help or with difficulties or young people with mobility problems. These might include those with progressive neurological conditions, the various forms of arthritis and those with developmental problems. It might be used as a short-term assistive device as it is easily inserted and removed from a home.

The assistive device was deemed to be less clumsy than a stair lift but still large and invasive for a private home. The perceived size of the device and the consequent need for a larger staircase was a limitation noted by a number of subjects. Noise from the ratchet mechanism was a problem but one that was tolerated by this group, largely because they were aware that this was a prototype. This issue would need to be addressed before the device could be marketed.

It is important to note these results with care. While they certainly indicate that the subjects found the device useful it may be that some were reluctant to express negative views. Care was taken to ensure subjects knew that both negative and positive feedback would be useful about it and to ensure the interviews were not in earshot of the rest of the team of researchers; the interviewers did not participate in the ascent or descent of the stairs. However, it was clear to the subjects that the interviewers were part of the general research team – and this may have biased the results. Other research (Marcus and Schütz, 2005) has indicated that satisfaction surveys and feedback in general are often biased to the positive – and this is especially so with the elderly.

The professionals involved in the design and testing of the device were far more accepting of it than the volunteers who were interviewed. However, they did see a few aspects that the potential users did not. The authors are aware the volunteers only had a very short time to test, think about and respond to the new device. However, this paper is a practical example of how necessary the opinions of all the stakeholders are in the process of designing assistive technology, but most essential are those of the potential user. While the biomechanical and clinical results were very encouraging regarding the physical ability and safety of the use of the device, the results from the interviews had the last word as to the direction of the next stage of the project. The final conclusion is that some elements of design are worth keeping, but to make a truly functional and acceptable product major design changes still have to be made, especially regarding noise, stiffness and aesthetics. Funding is being sought to continue to develop this device.

13.7 References

Department of Trade and Industry and Metra Martech Limited (2003) Avoiding slips, trips and broken hips. Falls on stairs in the home involving older people. Statistics. Available at: http://www.dti.gov.uk/homesafetynetwork/pdffalls/stats2.pdf

Hill LD, Haslam RA, Howarth PA, Brooke-Wavell K, Sloane JE (2000) Safety of older people on stairs: behavioural factors. Loughborough University, UK

Marcus B, Schütz A (2005) Who are the people reluctant to participate in research? Personality correlates of four different types of nonresponse as inferred by self- and observer ratings. Journal of Personality 73: 959–984

McCreadie C, Seale J, Tinker A, Turner-Smith A (2002) Older people and mobility in the home: in search of useful assistive technologies. The British Journal of Occupational Therapy 65: 54–60

Seale J, McCreadie C, Turner-Smith A, Tinker A (2002) Older people as partners in assistive technology research: the use of focus groups in the design process. Technology and Disability 14: 21–29

Shimada H, Uchiyama Y, Kakurai S (2003) Specific effects of balance and gait exercises on physical function among the frail elderly. Clinical Rehabilitation 17: 72–479

Steffen TM, Hacker TA, Mollinger L (2002) Age- and gender-related test performance in community-dwelling elderly people: six minute walk test, Berg Balance Scale, timed up and go test and gait speeds. Physical Therapy 82: 128–137

Chapter 14

The SMART Project: A User Led Approach to Developing Applications for Domiciliary Stroke Rehabilitation

G.A. Mountain, P.M. Ware, J. Hammerton, S.J. Mawson, H. Zheng, R. Davies, N. Black, H. Zhou, H. Hu, N. Harris and C. Eccleston

14.1 Introduction

The Smart Consortium is one of the five research groups funded under the EQUAL4 funding stream of the UK Engineering and Physical Sciences Research Council. It is a partnership of four universities, one industrial motion tracking company and one voluntary sector organisation, the Stroke Association. Membership includes academics in the field of occupational and physiotherapy, psychology, engineering, informatics, medical physics, design and those able to advocate on behalf of people with stroke. The researchers are advised by an expert panel of national and international academics. An expert group of people with strokes and their carers are consulted about any proposed project outputs.

The project, now in its third and final year, has been examining the appropriateness and effectiveness of technology to support stroke rehabilitation. Details of the overall work plan and progress can be found on the project web-site; http://hsc.shu.ac.uk/smart/.

14.2 Background

Stroke is the biggest cause of severe disability in the UK. Ten thousand people each year experience a first stroke, and another 3 000 have a further stroke (Stroke Association, 2001). The majority of people who sustain a stroke are elderly. They may have been in good health previously and managing independently but following the stroke can find themselves suddenly hospitalised or receiving hospital services at home, with subsequent needs for rehabilitation and lifestyle adjustments.

There is strong evidence that organised stroke care improves outcomes (Stroke Unit Trialists' Collaboration, 2005). Rehabilitation should commence as soon as possible after the stroke (Intercollegiate Working Party, 1999). However, active rehabilitation and advice is beneficial at all stages of the care pathway (Forster and Young, 2002). The National Service Framework for Older People recommends that rehabilitation should continue until maximum recovery has been achieved (DoH, 2001a). However, organisational issues and resource limitations can militate against access to services; nationally only 36% of patients admitted to hospital spend time on a stroke unit (RCP, 2002). There are also significant differences in the availability of specialist stroke services. In some locations, provision is reportedly basic, with rehabilitation being targeted solely at discharge from hospital and with little monitoring following return home (Tyson and Turner, 2000; Rudd *et al.*, 2001). Interviews with people who have experienced stroke confirmed a lack of satisfaction with rehabilitation services and a desire (or unmet need) for more directed rehabilitation in the critical period immediately post discharge (Pound *et al.*, 1998; Stroke Association, 2001). Consequently, there is important research developing technologies to encourage stroke rehabilitation with a variety of intelligent engineering solutions in the home (Bradley *et al.*, 2004), and also in a clinical environment (Hawkins *et al.*, 2002).

A systematic review of literature on user acceptance and satisfaction with assistive rehabilitation technology was undertaken in the early stages of the SMART project. The aim of the review was to inform the engineering team developing the assistive rehabilitation device. There was a lack of published research specifically on the user's perspective on the practicalities of such devices in the home, or the psycho-social effects of home based rehabilitation intervention devices. Studies of assistive technology in general terms underlined the importance of incorporating users' views at an early stage in the design and development process. Unless devices meet the needs of users in terms of outcomes and usability they will not ultimately be used clinically. Moreover, a major aspect of current government policy in reforming the NHS emphasises the involvement of service users in the development of services and as active participants in research (DoH, 2000; Hanley *et al.*, 2004).

14.3 The SMART Project

The project considers how home based rehabilitation interventions for stroke rehabilitation can be promoted through the use of advanced sensor technology and a computerised decision interface. The aim is for stroke patients at home to carry out exercises and activities that can be observed and measured both by the patients themselves and remotely by clinicians. Patients will receive feedback on their performance through the screen based information and display as well as through electronic messages from health care professionals. (Figure 14.1 sets out the system architecture.)

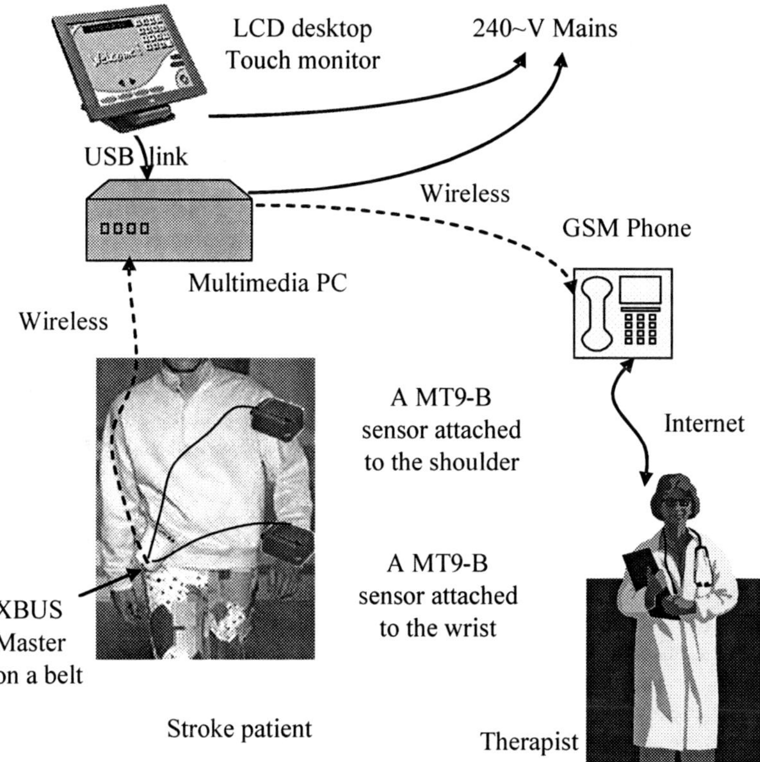

Figure 14.1. Architecture of the SMART system

Seven stroke specialist therapists from our two sites in Wiltshire and Sheffield, in both acute and primary care, met researchers to advise on appropriate movements on which to focus. The interventions we have targeted for rehabilitation were those identified by these therapists as being the most important and fundamental to independence, namely sit to stand/stand to sit; and reach out and grasp with the upper limb. To date the project has concentrated upon the upper limb movement as this tends to be relatively neglected in favour of lower limb rehabilitation and transfer abilities. The focus on enabling patients to return home has meant an understandable early emphasis on lower limb movement to ensure weight bearing and mobility.

One of the initial tasks of the project was to undertake an analysis of the functional movement patterns. Normative age matched data was unavailable so stroke and non-stroke participants were included. Each movement was recorded using the Codamotion 3D movement analysis system (Charnwood Dynamics Ltd) and kinematic parameters were measured and analysed. Through this we were able to identify key abnormalities in the stroke subjects' movements that were clinically significant and could be focused on by our device. Inertial sensor technology using

MT9 and Xbus equipment (Xsens Technologies B.V., The Netherlands) has been used to track the limb movement, ensuring that the sensors are able to accurately reflect the necessary range and quality of movement identified through previous work and necessary for clinical requirements (Zheng *et al.,* 2005a; Zhou and Hu, 2005). An important aspect of the work has been ensuring that information provided to users is of value to them and that the visual representation is lifelike and understandable. To this end the data from the sensors is translated into the presentation of a rendered limb. The movement undertaken by the person wearing the sensors is then represented through an Internet based or digital decision interface screen. Information can be provided to the wearer *in situ* and to a practitioner based at a remote location. Information in a different format to that for users is given to the health care professionals (Zheng *et al.,* 2005b). Separate focus groups of therapists and health care professionals have assisted with identifying what information is needed to ensure safe and effective clinical decision making. We are now at the stage where the prototype technological devices for upper limb movement and for the computerised decision interface have been developed.

14.4 Methods of User Consultation

At an early stage in the project we conducted a one-off consultation with separate groups of users of stroke services, carers of people with stroke and professionals in different locations to the project field work areas (McNair *et al.*, 2004). Participants were recruited by the Family Support Officers from the Stroke Association who were also present at the groups to assist the research facilitator and support the participants. The purpose was to identify the sorts of issues that are important to users so that they could be built into the development and testing of our devices. We set out to investigate what users and carers thought would be a useful role for a technology to assist in rehabilitation and what outcomes they would like from such a device. We sought their opinions on usability and any design ideas that they generated. We were also keen to elicit user and carer views on remote monitoring of patients' use of the device and subsequent progress. We asked for users' and carers' ideas as to what they foresaw as possible problems for the use of a device in their home. The group interviews were taped and transcribed and the analysis was conducted according to the 'framework' method described by Lacey and Luff (2001). In this phase of the consultation fifteen users and carers participated in four separate focus groups.

In these groups the idea of a technological device for rehabilitation was welcomed and no reservations were expressed about the acceptability of the overall idea. Stroke patients were unanimous in seeing a device as a way of enabling them to get more help with rehabilitation. They were particularly impressed with the proposition that they would get quantifiable and objective feedback on their performance from a machine rather than praise from the physiotherapist. Both carers and users felt that the device could help them maintain their motivation by seeing concrete measurement of any changes in their ability to move correctly.

Although it was recognised that different people would have different needs, the need most frequently expressed was for help to improve upper limb functioning.

The key points that emerged across the first set of focus groups was that any technological devices should be:

- compact, simple to operate (and maintained by staff in the event of problems);
- usable by stroke patients preferably without the help of the carer, to encourage independence;
- available alongside the work of health professionals/physiotherapists (not replacing them);
- able to give encouraging feedback to patients about outcomes even when progress is slow.

These initial groups were generic in focus, as we had not at that stage developed specific technologies to demonstrate to the participants. The findings from these groups influenced the development of the prototype device.

Once we had developed a prototype we started the second phase of user and carer consultation by convening further groups to give detailed feedback on the actual devices. (Professionals were consulted separately over specific aspects of the technology and in particular the questions that should be asked through the decision support interface). At this stage we wanted to show the sensor equipment which would be attached to stroke patients as well as demonstrate the computer interface which was to give feedback to the user. We planned to use the resulting information from the focus groups to refine the equipment ready for testing with users at home. These clinical tests will form the third phase of the user consultation.

As the concept of remote monitoring and movement tracking is complicated we chose to have a series of focus groups with the same group of users and carers. In this way we could build up understanding of the various elements of the project rather than expect participants to conceptualise the different parts all at once. Thus we developed an expert group of users as promoted by recent DoH policy (DoH, 2001b). Many of them had already been involved in other aspects of the project concerned with measurement and analysis of movement pattern data and were in some way familiar with the ideas behind the project. We met with the users and carers on three separate occasions; ten people with stroke and six carers were consulted in total for this second phase.

At the initial consultation group in this phase, users were introduced to the project background and aims and the types of technology to be utilised. They were encouraged to raise questions and seek clarification. Subsequent groups with the same participants have considered both the wearable device bearing the movement sensor technology and the screen based decision support interface. At this stage we had a number of different attachment methods for the devices prepared by design colleagues using dummy prototype movement sensors. Participants were encouraged to handle and try on the proposed technologies and give their opinions. Ease of handling, comfort in use, accuracy of positioning and visual acceptability were discussed which resulted in designers making further adjustments to test at the next group. Demonstrations of the decision support interface were provided, so that users could view the screen interface and again provide their feedback. Types of feedback both visual and auditory were demonstrated and participants made suggestions about measures to be used to assess progress.

Informatics, physiotherapy experts and designers have accompanied these groups to respond to users' comments. The groups were taped and transcribed and the user group trying the attachment devices with the dummy movement sensors was videotaped. This enabled not only analysis of the verbal feedback but also the capture of the movements of people with stroke as they handled the devices and attempted to position them correctly. Stroke people formed one set of users whilst their carers formed another group so as to allow their different perspectives to be articulated.

One of the informatics experts was also affected by a stroke and he was able to attend both the user focus groups and the health professionals consultation group for the decision support interface enabling a fuller appreciation of different stakeholders views.

Further refinements to the devices and the digital interface are to be made following the response at these groups, and this will lead into the third stage of user consultation which will consist of clinical tests of the system in the homes of people who have had a stroke.

14.5 Results of the Consultation

Our first phase of consultation took place before we had any prototypes to demonstrate and so we were able to develop the technology in accordance with the principles that emerged from these initial groups *i.e.* a compact technology that would be simple to operate and maintain, to be used as independently as possible by the patient, that would work alongside health professionals and that would encourage perseverance and motivation through clear feedback to patients. Our second phase of consultation has given us feedback on our prototypes for the computer interface and the sensor attachments.

In trying out the different methods of attaching the sensors we have had to reduce some of the flexibility initially built into the design. For example, to accommodate both right and left sided stroke related weakness we initially incorporated a clip that could allow right or left handed use. However, in demonstrating this to users and getting their feedback it became clear that having this flexibility was confusing to patients. It was important that the device could simply and obviously be attached without having to work out which clip could be undone.

We were also able to narrow down the type of fastening that could be used easily. Some of the connections required two hands to be used to hold the device in place, which for stroke patients without normal use of one arm was impractical and would lead to dependence on carers to wear the equipment. Other fastening using Velcro material involved too much friction for the device to maintain its correct position. By having users try on the different styles of attachment we were able to see for ourselves how the sensor was positioned and relate this to users' perception of comfort and recognition of the correct placement.

We found that by enabling users to put the devices on and off several times and wear them for short periods we were able to understand whether initial manoeuvres could be learnt easily. One of the attachment methods used a long strap to be fastened around the chest to keep the sensor in place. Although there was initial confusion as to how to place the strap, users found that once they understood the concept and could see how it worked in practice they overcame their doubts and considered that it was an easy and wearable option. Another option was a less complicated rigid attachment that appeared simpler to put on, but users commented that the rigidity reduced the comfort although they appreciated the simplicity. Another option to attach the sensors was in the form of a sleeve which the user slid on to the affected arm. Although this appeared simpler, being all in one (rather than separate shoulder and wrist attachments) we found it was difficult for one size to fit all users. It also proved to be more difficult for users to position correctly.

The device has to be connected to the power source and there were different options to consider as to how the sensors could be wired to the battery. By trying out the equipment both with fixed and with removable wires, we were able to assess which was easier to handle and apply. Initial reactions of concern were not always borne out once the device had been handled and worn.

The computer screen interface which shows the user's arm movement and provides feedback on progress and communicates with remote clinicians was also demonstrated to the groups. Initial findings from these groups suggest that even those older users who have little or no experience of home computers are able to provide useful feedback on what they would find helpful. Lack of familiarity with information technology did not prevent engagement with the issues. New ideas were generated about different ways of feeding back information to users.

Using data from the templates of both normal and stroke affected movement, participants were able to see the differences between the two movement trajectories. Surprise was expressed at how great the difference was, once seen on screen, suggesting that patients are not fully aware of the adjustments they make to compensate for loss of muscle tone. The visual presentation of this difference in movement may enable users to appreciate more clearly what therapists are working towards and may enable them to focus on particular sections of the movement of which they were previously unaware.

We were able to check with users the sorts of information that they would find helpful in understanding their progress (or lack of it). They were interested in a measure which rated how close their movement was to a target movement of a normal arm. They were also interested in the display of their previous attempts at the exercises on screen to demonstrate both where they were coming from as well as to see what they were trying to achieve. Users suggested that the screen could be customised for each user depending on what level of display they might find helpful. This could extend to the way the colours and size of text were shown. They appreciated the ability to 'see' their movements from a variety of different angles such as a birds-eye view, side or front view.

We also gained useful feedback on the interactive nature of the system. Users and carers expressed their interest in being able to make their own notes to explain differences in performance. Fluctuations in the ability to perform exercises could then be explained by events such as having a cold or having fallen which would enable therapists and users alike to interpret the data more intelligently. Users were also keen to be able to access their movement history together with notes made in earlier stages of rehabilitation. They felt that this record of information and subsequent written dialogue with health care professionals would give them a sense of control and empowerment within the rehabilitation process.

Participants were asked their opinions about the idea of remote monitoring and the questions that would be asked of users before they started their programme for each session. They were reassured by the questions about their health and comfortable about information from the privacy of their homes being sent to clinicians in a health care setting. They recognised that clinicians were not available whenever they were using the equipment but were interested in the idea of having fixed times when professionals might be able to interact with them in real time.

We sought more detailed feedback from users as to their understanding of the questions the system would ask each user to ensure that exercise was safe. We were able to explore questions about general tiredness and more specific tightness of limbs to find a balance between overprotecting users on the one hand and allowing them to do too much movement when it might be detrimental.

14.6 Discussion

The SMART project is developing new rehabilitation technology that has not been tried before. At this stage in the development we are working on ‘proof of concept’ ideas. We want to ensure that the technology works and gives reliable and accurate information on patient movement. However, it is important to build in user views at this early stage rather than wait until the technology is proven. We are looking at each stage for confirmation or otherwise that what professionals, engineers and designers consider important is useful for patients and carers. Small decisions made at early stages may prevent or enable developments in the future. Ideas generated by users and carers may bring new perspectives on what is possible. Issues of comfort, wearability, attractiveness and usefulness all have a bearing on whether users and carers will actually use new technologies in practice. Therapists of various kinds are well aware of unused equipment stored in cupboards or used for entirely other purposes because users either did not see the point or found equipment too unpleasant to use. We are therefore keen to consult with users at different stages in this project to ensure as far as possible that the effort and resources put into major research projects such as this will have a good chance of usefulness and acceptability. The discipline of involving designers at an early stage has demonstrated the importance of checking what is possible before the decisions are made that rule out desired options.

The users and carers we have consulted were well motivated and keen to participate. The numbers of users were limited in order that we could explain the project concepts. Our work with this group has enabled us to develop our understanding together of how the project can progress and they are keen to be involved with the testing of the final versions of the devices. In this way we are developing an expert patient group who can influence the shape of the project as it progresses. The experience emphasises the importance of consultation with all stakeholders at regular stages of the project. More data about how the system operates in the home environment will be available after the full user trials in 2006.

14.7 Acknowledgements

The research is funded by EPSRC under the EQUAL4 programme. The authors wish to acknowledge the work done by Bardie McNair and Nargis Islam in the initial stage of consultation with users and carers, and Marianne Gittoes who undertook analysis of the movement templates.

14.8 References

Bradley DA, Hawley MS, Enderby PM, Brownsell SJ, Mawson SJ *et al.* (2004) Remote rehabilitation using an intelligent exoskeleton. In: Proceedings of CWUAAT'04, Cambridge, UK

Charnwood Dynamics Ltd., Unit 2 Victoria Mills, Fowke Street, Rothley, Leicestershire LE7 7PJ, UK. Available at: http://www.codamotion.com/

DoH (2000) The NHS plan: a plan for investment, a plan for reform. Department of Health, London, UK

DoH (2001a) National service framework for older people. Department of Health, London, UK

DoH (2001b) The expert patient: a new approach to chronic disease management for the 21st century. Department of Health, London, UK

Forster A, Young J (2002) Clinical and cost effectiveness of physiotherapy in the management of elderly people following stroke. Chartered Society of Physiotherapists, London, UK

Hanley B, Bradburn J, Barnes M, Evans C, Goodare H *et al.* (2004) Involving the public in NHS, public health and social care research: briefing notes for researchers. Involve. Available at: http://www.invo.org.uk/

Hawkins P, Smith J, Alcock S, Topping M, Harwin W, Loureiro R *et al.* (2002) GENTLE/S project: design and ergonomics of a stroke rehabilitation system. In: Proceedings of CWUAAT'02, Cambridge, UK

Lacey A, Luff D (2001) Qualitative data analysis. Trent Focus Group, UK

McNair B, Islam N, Eccleston C, Mountain G, Harris N (2004) EPSRC smart rehabilitation: technological applications for use in the home by people who have had a stroke and their primary carers. Report of a focus group study. University of Bath and the Royal National Hospital for Rheumatic diseases NHS Trust and Sheffield Hallam University. Unpublished paper

Pound P, Gompertez P, Ebrahim S (1998) A patient-centred study of the consequences of stroke. Clinical Rehabilitation 12(4): 338–347

RCP (2002) Summary report on the national sentinel stroke audit 2001–2. Royal College of Physicians, UK

Rudd AG, Irwin P, Rutledge Z, Lowe D, Wade DT *et al.* (2001) Regional variations in stroke care in England, Wales and Northern Ireland: results from the National Sentinel Audit of Stroke. Clinical Rehabilitation 15: 562–572

Stroke Unit Trialists' Collaboration (2005) Organised inpatient (stroke unit) care for stroke. The Cochrane Database of Systematic Reviews 2005, Issue 4, John Wiley, Chichester, UK. Available at: http://www.cochrane.org/index0.htm

The Stroke Association (2001) Speaking out about stroke services. The Stroke Association, London, UK

Tyson S, Turner G (2000) Discharge and follow-up for people with stroke: what happens and why. Clinical Rehabilitation 14: 381–392

Xsens Technologies B.V., Capitool 50, Postbus 545, 7500 A M Enschede, The Netherlands. Available at: http://www.xsens.com

Zheng H, Black ND, Harris N (2005a) Position-sensing technologies for movement analysis in stroke rehabilitation. Medical and Biological Engineering and Computing 43(4): 413–420

Zheng H, Davies R, Black ND (2005b) Web-based monitoring system for home-based rehabilitation with stroke patients. In: Proceedings of the 18th IEEE Symposium on Computer-based Medical System, Dublin, Ireland

Zhou H, Hu H (2005) Inertial motion tracking of human arm movements in home-based rehabilitation. In: Proceedings of the IEEE International Conference on Mechatronics and Automation, Ontario, Canada

Chapter 15

Non-speech Operated Emulation of Keyboard

A.J. Sporka, S.H. Kurniawan and P. Slavík

15.1 Introduction

Assistive technologies have recently received a lot of well-deserved attention. These technologies allow the adaptation of computing equipment's interfaces to users' special needs, and thus help the users to reduce social barriers produced by their impairment.

A specific group of impaired users are people with motor disabilities, who face significant difficulties when using standard keyboards and mice. Usually, a dedicated piece of hardware is used to compensate for such disabilities, when they become severe. This type of hardware can include different breath switches (sip-and-puff controllers) or eye trackers. These devices have been extensively investigated in recent literature as means of user interface control.

One solution for people with severe motor impairments is speech recognition technology. Currently, this technology is employed as a means of controlling various telephony applications (such as phone number or flight information inquiries) or devices in hands-busy situations (*e.g.* operating cellular telephones while driving). Speech recognition has recently also been employed as an alternative means of general user interface control or text input operations, thus relieving users of the need to use keyboards.

Some of the most important features of the speech control—and acoustic control in general—are its low cost and its easy deployment on various platforms. However, some forms of severe motor impairment (*e.g.*, cerebral palsy) are frequently accompanied by speech disorders, posing substantial problems to even state-of-art speech recognizers. It is not unusual for the acoustic abilities of such people to be limited only to humming or hissing, or similar non-speech sounds, which render the speech recognition techniques, in principle, unusable.

Until recently the use of non-speech sounds for control of computers remained only of marginal interest to the HCI community. Previous work is limited to a few isolated projects, such as Igarashi and Hughes, 2001, where non-speech sounds are used as an extension of the speech-based interaction with the TV remote control, or

Hämäläinen *et al.* (2004) where the non-speech sounds are used to control computer games.

Recently, two systems for non-speech acoustic control of the mouse pointer have emerged. Sporka, Kurniawan and Slavík (2004) proposed and successfully tested a system where a mouse cursor was operated by producing specific melodies of whistling or humming. Using these, the mouse cursor was steered along either *x*- or *y*-axis at one time. Bilmes *et al.* (2005) proposed to use chanting for similar purposes. In their system, the pitch of voice is used to steer the velocity of the cursor while the type of vowel sound ("ahh", "eyy", "eee" ...) specifies the direction of movement. These two instances represent non-speech control systems, where the pitch or timbre of a tone is used as a metaphor of analogue geometric data: The parameters of tones are directly mapped to the velocity vector of the mouse cursor.

It is however possible to define a system of acoustic gestures (*e.g.* short melodies, or rhythmic patterns), in which each gesture is associated with one elementary command or action that is triggered immediately after completion of the gesture. Such a use scenario is suitable for interaction by means of discrete events, such as letter-by-letter input of text, which is a common paradigm of keyboard use.

This is the focus of our paper; here we describe the use of the non-speech sounds for entering text by means of keyboard emulation. A solution to this problem has existed for more than 150 years in the form of the well-known Morse code (the work of Morse and Vail in 1835). Morse may indeed be produced with non-speech sounds and interpreted by the computer as the means of keyboard emulation. In Morse code, the information is encoded only in length of beeps and pauses in between.

While respecting this classical form of communication, we have defined two alternative "non-speech alphabets" comprised of acoustic gestures involving also the melody of their elementary tones.

The goal of this study is to investigate the efficiency and user acceptance of the three methods mentioned in typing short segments of text (such as short instant messages, or search queries on web pages). This application was considered the most suitable for the methods discussed.

15.2 The Input Methods

All methods described in this paper are based on the analysis of tone sequences generated by the user that comprise individual acoustic gestures. The gestures are matched with those previously assigned to different keys. Whenever a match is found, the appropriate keystroke is emulated. The users then receive the visual feedback of their input to the system. The system overview common for all methods is shown in Figure 15.1.

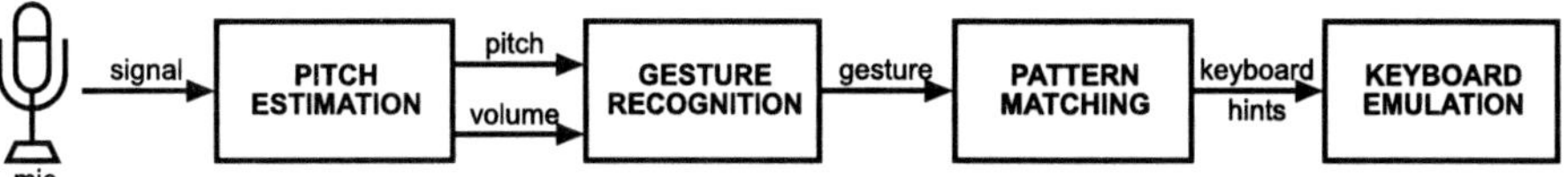

Figure 15.1. The method overview

In our recent work (Sporka *et al.*, 2005) we have compared the usability of different types of non-verbal sound that the humans are capable of, especially the humming, whistling, and voiceless fricative sounds. These are parameterized with a pitch that is deliberately controlled by the tension of the vocal chord, or the volume of the oral cavity. The general users' preference was towards humming, which we have decided to employ in our methods.

To track voice pitch a simple estimation method of basic voice frequency f_0, based on the autocorrelation, has been used.

In our research, we compare the efficiency of three different sets of non-speech patterns, the classic Morse code and the following two new non-speech input methods that we have designed.

- *Pitch-to-address mapping*, where the pitch of each of the flat tones in a sequence determines the address (the coordinates) of a key in discrete space. This mapping is based on generation of tones of absolute pitch.
- *Pattern-to-key mapping*, where each key to be emulated is assigned a sequence of tonal primitives (flat tone, raising tone, falling tone, and pause).

The prototypes of all the methods mentioned in this text were implemented as standalone applications for the win32 environment in MS VC++ 6.0 and are available for download on the U3I project homepage (see references).

15.2.1 Pitch-to-address Mapping Method

This method is based on the interpretation of a sequence of tones produced by humming, as a vector of coordinates of keys in a keyboard layout. After the last tone is finished, the keystroke of the key located at the specified coordinates is emulated.

For the purposes of this method, a tone was defined as a signal produced by humming whose pitch is in a certain interval. These intervals do not overlap and may be calibrated to cover the range in which the humming has a comfortable pitch for a particular user's vocal tract.

There is a trade-off between the number of coordinates in the vector and the size of the set of tones. Considering the number of keys on standard keyboards, we decided to use a sequence of three tones, each one from the scale of four. This enables the addressing of 64 different keys, which is sufficient for the emulation of the most frequently used keys or their combinations. The actual coordinate space used for our method is shown in Figure 15.2. The first coordinate (A1) determines a row, the second one (A2) specifies a group of four keys, and the last one (A3) determines the key.

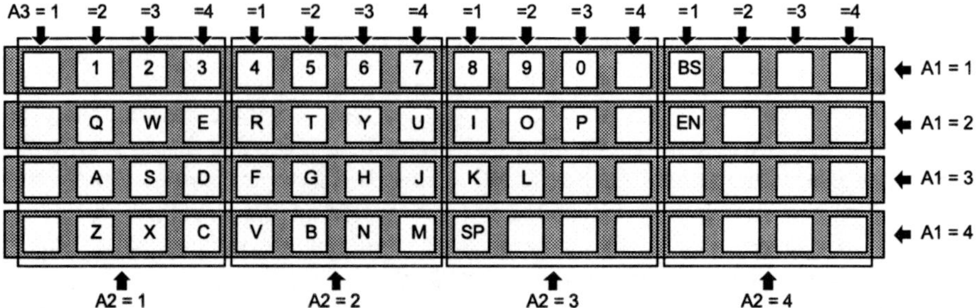

Figure 15.2. The address space of the keys for the pitch-to-address mapping method

For example,to type “CU”, the user has to hum a sequence of tones 4, 1, 4 (which produces “C”) and then 2, 2, 4 (which produces “U”). This example is also shown in Figure 15.3.

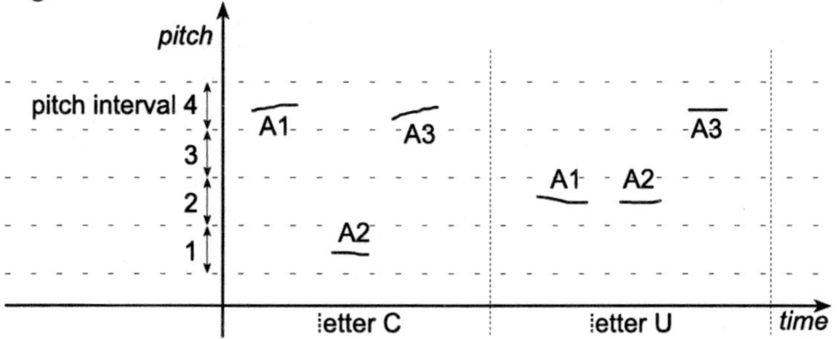

Figure 15.3. Melody of humming in the pitch-to-address mapping method to type “CU”

The on-screen representation of the virtual keyboard shows the current status of the system as well as the feedback to the tone the user hums. The entire keyboard is divided into four areas marked with different colours. While the user maintains a tone, the system emphasizes the colour of the area that has been assigned that tone. The area is selected when the tone stops. After that, the area gets divided into four equal sub-areas (as shown in Figure 15.4) and another tone may start, etc.

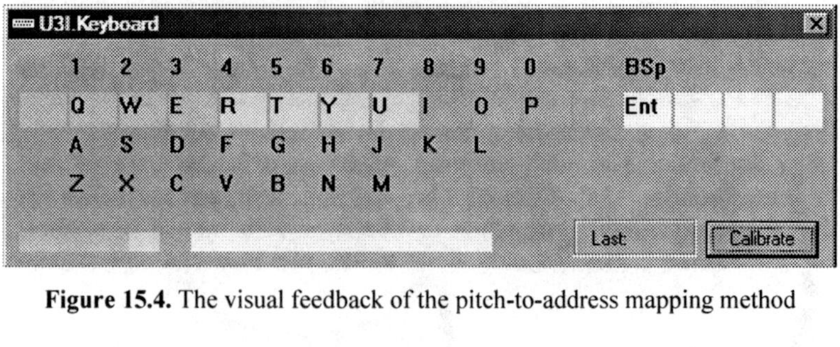

Figure 15.4. The visual feedback of the pitch-to-address mapping method

15.2.2 Pattern-to-key Mapping

This method is based on the recognition of the following four tonal pattern primitives, whose notation, used in this text, is shown in the brackets:

- Flat Tone
  - Low or High (symbols _ and ¯)
  - Short or Long (symbols _ and __)
- Raising tone (symbol /)
- Falling tone (symbol \)
- Pause (shown as a discontinuation of the pattern)

We have defined the tonal pattern as the sequence of the tonal primitives that follows these rules:

- A flat tone in a pattern is preceded and/or followed by a pause unless being the first or the last primitive in the pattern.
- A raising tone in a pattern may be preceded or followed by a falling tone (and vice versa) without a pause between them.
- To overcome the need for the user's absolute pitch hearing, the pitch of the tone is resolved only if there is either a raising or a falling tone or if there is more than one flat tone of differing pitches.
- Pause never occurs at the beginning or at the end of a pattern.

Using these rules, we developed an alphabet of acoustic gestures. We considered the frequency distribution of the letters in English text as mentioned in Beker and Piper, 1982, so that the most frequent characters are assigned the simplest gestures (E, I, T, etc.).

The window of the application shows the table of gestures organized alphabetically or to reflect the standard QWERTY layout (see Figure 15.5). Each field of the table contains the label of the key and its respective gesture. After the user successfully produces a gesture, the field with the corresponding character flashes, the keystroke is emulated, and the last recognized gesture appears in the box labelled Input pattern.

15.2.3 Morse Code

Morse code recognition was implemented by making simplification to the pattern-to-key mapping option by defining patterns where only flat tones were considered.

We have used a standard International Morse Code (IMC) with explicit definition of *space* ("–...–"; *double-dash* in IMC) and *backspace* characters ("......"; *error* in the IMC).

The visual feedback for this method has been adjusted to show the Morse code patterns rather than pattern-to-key assignments, as shown in Figure 15.6.

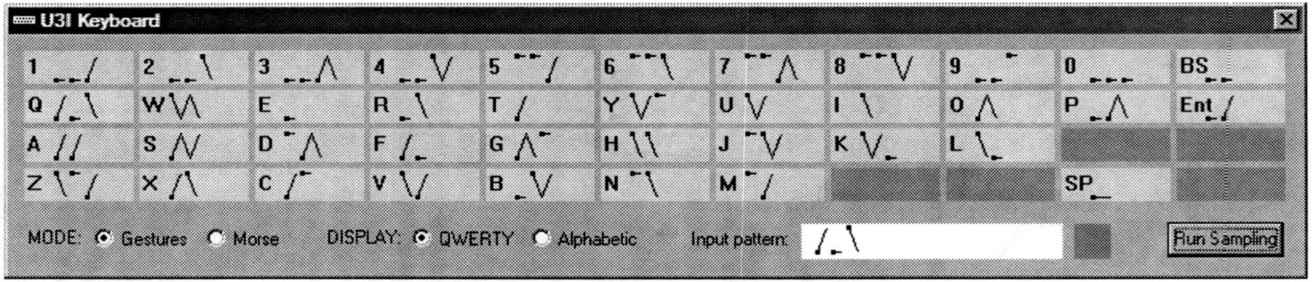

Figure 15.5. The user interface of the system, showing the assignment of the non-speech patterns to the keys of the keyboard

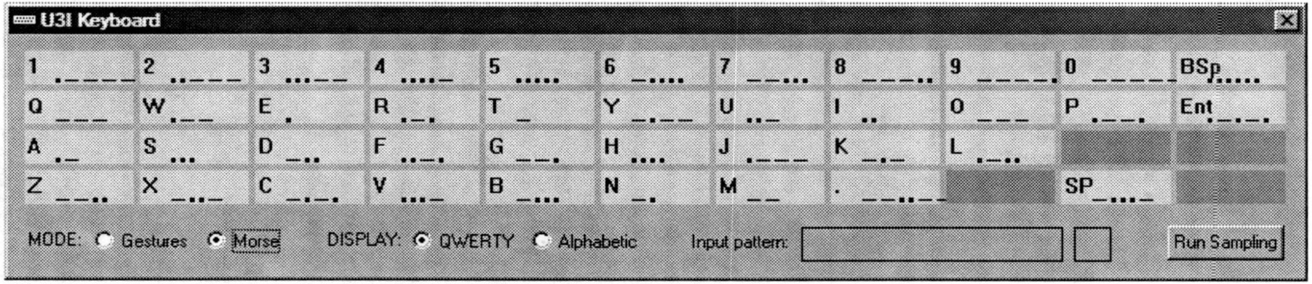

Figure 15.6. The user interface in the Morse-code mode

15.3 User Study

The hypothesis of this study was that the pitch-to-address and pattern-to-key mappings would be easier-to-use than the Morse code. We also expected that the pitch-to-address technique would gain from its intuitiveness and the pattern-to-key mapping would take less time than the Morse code as its patterns are shorter on average.

The designed methods were tested by nine regular computer users (defined as people who use computers at least 5 hours a week), aged 19-28, 3 females and 6 males university students, either at postgraduate or undergraduate levels. The participants were asked to write 4 sentences (all containing 11 characters including spaces). All participants either had no visual impairment or wore corrective lenses at the time of the experiment. A Pentium-4 1.7 GHz PC running Windows XP with a 17" monitor set at 1024 by 768 pixels resolution was used. Each participant tested the system in a quiet room accompanied only by the experimenter. To minimize the noise interference from the surrounding environment, the participants wore headsets throughout the sessions. Participants' interactions with the software were recorded using Camtasia Studio 2 screen capture software.

At the beginning of each session the experimenter informed the participants that the purpose of the study was to investigate how easy it was for them to type two sentences through vocal sounds and not to measure their performance in using the system. The experimenter then introduced the participant to the system by playing a series of demonstration MP3 files containing the examples of the input for different modes. The participants were then given 5 minutes to try each mode after being reminded that the system was sensitive to noise. They were also informed that they were allowed to take as many breaks as they wished, either between modes or between characters.

The sequence of the tested modes was order balanced as much as possible. Table 15.1 describes the sequence that each participant went through (Px indicates participant ID).

Table 15.1. The user study organistion

Sentences	**P1, P7**	**P2, P6**	**P3, P8, P5**	**P4, P9**
"HOW ARE YOU"	Morse alphabetic	Pattern-to-key QWERTY	Pitch-to-address	Morse QWERTY
"WHERE TO GO"	Pattern-to-key QWERTY	Pitch-to-address	Morse QWERTY	Pattern-to-key alphabetic
"I WAIT HERE"	Pitch-to-address	Morse alphabetic	Pattern-to-key alphabetic	Pitch-to-address
"HE IS ANGRY"	Morse QWERTY	Pattern-to-key alphabetic	Morse alphabetic	Pattern-to-key QWERTY

15.3.1 Results

Because there were only nine participants, a strong conclusion based on statistical analysis could not be performed. However, the results indicate quite a strong trend. In ranking the modes, all users but one were in agreement that Morse QWERTY was the easiest to use and the most preferred (the remaining participant chose Morse alphabetic). Seven users disliked the pitch-to-address mapping keyboard the most (the other two disliked the pattern-to-key alphabetic and pattern-to-key QWERTY, respectively). The computer log shows that the Morse code was also the fastest to finish. The average times of the nine users to finish a sentence are shown in Table 15.2.

The users reported certain difficulties with humming the required acoustic patterns for the pattern-to-key and pitch-to-address methods. This may suggest that while the pitch of the tone in the non-verbal input is a useful and intuitive means of the continuous data input (*e.g.* for the control of the mouse pointer, as discussed in section *Overview*), its advantages for text input are not that strong.

Participants were also asked to comment on their preference, complaints, opinions, etc, regarding each mode. Some users felt that they could not inflect their voice to match the inflection required by the Pattern-to-key keyboard. All but one said that QWERTY arrangement was easier to operate than alphabetical one. Two users did not make any mistake while typing the requested 4 sentences. The rest made between 1-7 errors requiring backspace (the Pattern-to-key keyboard produced the most number of errors across all participants). Interestingly, even though the pitch-to-address keyboard was the one disliked by the most participants, it was the one mode where all users made no errors.

It was noticeable that after 3-4 characters, users took longer pauses. In general, users stated that they like the system (especially the Morse keyboard) and think that it would be easy to master. In conclusion, the small user study that we performed, indicate that all the modes are usable and receive quite positive user opinion to a certain extent.

Table 15.2. The user study results

Method	**Completion time [s]**	**Type rate [char./min]**	**Number of errors**
Morse alphabetic	42 ± 4	16 ± 1.5	3 ± 1
Morse QWERTY	40 ± 4	16.5 ± 1.5	3 ± 2
Pattern-to-key alphabetic	54 ± 6	12 ± 1.5	5 ± 2
Pattern-to-key QWERTY	47 ± 4	14 ± 1	4 ± 3
Pitch-to-address mode	45 ± 5	15 ± 2	0

15.4 Conclusions

From the results of the usability study, we may conclude that all users participating were able to finish the task with any of the three methods we have introduced (pitch-to-address, pattern-to-key, and Morse).

While the average completion times were comparable for all methods, all users felt more confident and completed faster when using the Morse code, but made less errors when using the pitch-to-address mapping. Considering the cost/acceptance of these three modes, we can conclude that the Morse code input method is still the best technique to operate a keyboard using non-speech sound. This is an interesting finding, because whereas the melody was a natural means of geometric data entry in the keyboard emulation it appears not as useful as the melody-free method, such as the Morse code input method.

The type rate of approximately 16 characters per minute is however comparable with other assistive techniques. For example, eye-dwell typing, as described by Hansen *et al.* (2003), reports a type rate of 16.5 char/min, which is still only a fraction of type rates commonly achievable on standard keyboards. Our expectation of our non-speech typing methods being suitable, especially for the typing of short texts, therefore proved realistic. Our future work will include an integration of these techniques with the acoustic control cursor for the mouse pointer to allow a transparent replacement of the mouse and keyboard devices. Potential use cases include instant messaging and operating web-based search engines.

Our immediate follow-up will be to perform a larger usability study that would yield larger amount of statistical data that would allow detailed comparison of the non-speech acoustic text input with other methods, such as eye tracking operated on-screen keyboard.

15.5 Acknowledgements

This research has been supported by Ministry of Education, Youth and Sports under research programme MSM6840770014 of the Czech Republic. The authors wish to thank Lidia Oshlyansky, University of Wales Swansea, for her help with proofreading of the text.

15.6 References

Beker H, Piper F (1982) Cipher systems. Wiley-Interscience, New York, USA

Bilmes JA, Li X, Malkin J, Kilanski K, Wright R *et al.* (2005) The vocal joystick: a voicebased human-computer interface for individuals with motor impairments. In: Proceedings of the Human Language Technology Conference, Vancouver, Canada

Hämäläinen P, Mäki-Patola T, Pulkki V, Airas M (2004) Musical computer games played by singing. In: Proceedings of the 7th International Conference on Digital Audio Effects, Naples, Italy

Hansen JP, Johansen AS, Hansen DW, Itoh K, Mashino S (2003) Command without a click: dwell time typing by mouse and gaze selections. In: Proceedings of INTERACT'03, Amsterdam, The Netherlands

Igarashi T, Hughes JF (2001) Voice as sound: using non-verbal voice input for interactive control. In: Proceedings of the 14th Annual ACM symposium on User Interface Software and Technology, New York, USA

Kitto KL (1993) Development of a low-cost Sip and Puff mouse. In: Proceedings of the 16th Annual Conference of RESNA, Las Vegas, USA

Liffick BW (2003) Assistive technology in computer science. In: Proceedings of the 1st International Symposium on Information and Communication Technologies, Dublin, Ireland

Sibert LE, Jacob RJK (2000) Evaluation of eye gaze interaction. In: Proceedings of the CHI'00, The Hague, The Netherlands

Sporka AJ, Kurniawan SH, Slavík P, Mahud M (2005) Tonal control of mouse cursor (U^3I): a usability study with the elderly. In: Proceedings of the HCI International 2005, Las Vegas, USA

Sporka AJ, Kurniawan SH, Slavík P (2004) Whistling user interface (U^3I). The 8th ERCIM International Workshop "User Interfaces For All", Vienna, Austria

Whistling User Interface. Project homepage, on-line resource. Available at: http:// www.u3i.info

Chapter 16

Dysarthric Speech Measures for Use in Evidence-based Speech Therapy

W.A. Simm, P.E. Roberts and M.J. Joyce

16.1 Introduction

The main aim of this research is to develop software to aid speech therapists in their work with dysarthric speakers. By producing indicators of speech quality and providing therapists with a way to objectively assess and monitor the therapy they can offer, dysarthric speakers may benefit from distinct and immediate feedback to promote recovery. This will promote the level of inclusion experienced by dysarthric speakers in society, and support the current trend towards evidence-based practice amongst health care professionals.

Dysarthria is one of the most common speech disorders and was selected for study here for this reason. It is a condition where the fundamental and conceptual communication and language faculties of the speaker are intact; the communication problem is caused by the actual articulation or production of the speech (Roberts, 2004). Given the increasing ageing population, the prevalence of dysarthria in the population is likely to increase because of the association.

Research is currently centred on investigating the differences in word closure between dysarthric and normal speakers. This paper presents these word closure differences as a new potential metric for the assessment of dysarthric speech. Two other prototype computer-based dynamic speech measures have also been produced. These measures have been designed to assist clinicians in their assessment and patients in the improvement of speech. The prototype measures comprise a novel rate/gap display and a novel cumulative frequency plot.

The two prototype measures, a rate/gaps display and cumulative formant plots, were first proposed by Roberts (2004), and furthered by Simm *et al.* (2005). Automatic analysis of word closure, as a potential metric for the assessment of dysarthric speech, was proposed by Simm *et al.* (2005). Other researchers in this field include Harel *et al.* (2004) who proposed changes in the variability of the first formant frequency of Parkinsonian speech as a potential biomarker of early disease progression. Research into the ageing effects on the first formant frequency of speech has been carried out by Max and Mueller (1996).

The background section of this paper briefly outlines how speech is produced, and introduces the dysarthric condition. It then introduces the previously documented prototype measures that are discussed in this paper. The paper then goes on to discuss current research into the analysis of word closure characteristics of dysarthric speakers and extends previous work. Samples from speakers with a variety of conditions that result in dysarthria are discussed.

16.2 Background

16.2.1 Speech Production

Human speech is produced by the vocal organs, which are identified in Figure 16.1. During speech production, air is forced out of the lungs, through the glottis between the vocal cords and the larynx to the three main cavities of the vocal tract. These cavities are the *pharynx* and the *oral* and *nasal* cavities. From here the air flow exits through the nose and mouth respectively (Lemmetty, 1999).

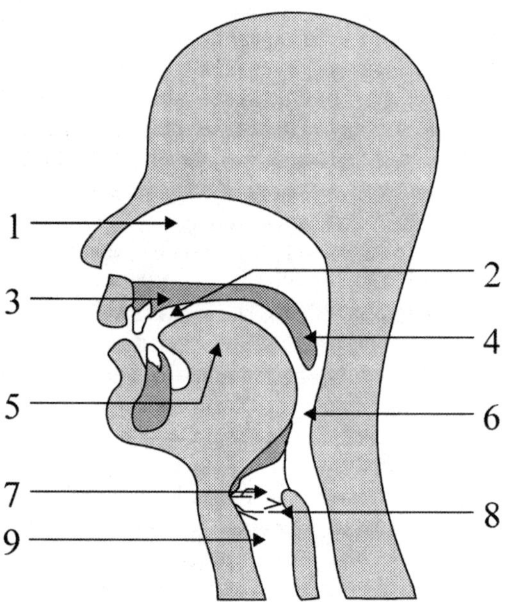

Figure 16.1. The human vocal organs: (1) Nasal cavity, (2) Oral cavity, (3) Hard Palate, (4) Uvula, (5) Tongue, (6) Pharynx, (7) Glottis, (8) Vocal cords, (9) Larynx

The glottis, which is the name given to the opening between the vocal chords, is the most important sound source in the speech system. The glottis modulates air flow by rapidly opening and closing, producing the sounds from which vowels and voiced consonants are produced (Lemmetty, 1999). When the glottis is open, the sounds that are produced are said to be voiced, and when closed any sounds produced are unvoiced (Laver, 1994).

16.2.2 Dysarthria

A speech disorder is defined as a "defect or abnormality that prevents an individual from communicating by means of spoken words" (NIDCH, 2004). Disorders are caused by hearing loss, neurological disorders, brain injury, drug abuse, physical impairments and vocal abuse, but often the cause is unknown.

Dysarthria is defined as a speech disorder resulting from paralysis, weakness or in-coordination of the speech musculature that is of neurological origin. A number of subsystems make up the speech system and in order for the speech produced to be clear, they must be coordinated with each other and work together. A motor disturbance in any one of respiratory, resonance, articulation or prosody systems can result in dysarthria. In adults, dysarthria can be caused by stroke, degenerative disease, infections, brain tumours, toxins, and other neurological conditions (Love and Webb, 1992).

Symptoms of dysarthria include slow, weak, imprecise or uncoordinated speech, generally referred to as "slurred". Dysarthric speakers can be misunderstood because listeners often pretend they have understood rather than suffer the embarrassment of asking the dysarthric speaker to repeat what they have said.

16.2.3 Speech Sample Collection

Speech samples were collected over a period of months from dysarthric speakers with a range of conditions including Parkinson's disease, Motor Neurone Disease and recovering stroke patients. Guidance in the selection of candidates and the supervision of sessions was undertaken by a Speech and Language Therapist (SLT) from the Morecambe Bay NHS Primary Care Trust. The procedure for collecting samples was to record set texts spoken by the client with a portable mini-disc recorder. The speech samples were then downloaded to computer via optical link for evaluation. The SLT was asked to evaluate and grade the speech, and to indicate any improvement in the client's speech if it was a return visit. Normal speech was also obtained for comparative purposes.

16.2.4 Prototype Speech Measures

The two prototype measures introduced previously include a rate/gaps display and a three-dimensional plot illustrating the two lowest formant frequencies of speech. The rate/gaps display and cumulative formant plots were first proposed by Roberts (2004) and furthered by Simm *et al.* (2005).

16.2.4.1 Rate/Gaps Display

Therapists currently exploit speech rate and the ratio between durations of utterances and silences. The rate/gaps display presents this information automatically in an easily interpreted way.

The premise to this measure was that dysarthria has particular effects on the prosody of the speech (Roberts, 2004). Prosody is the study of the characteristics of speech beyond the basic words and spectra, *e.g.* stress, intonation, tempo.

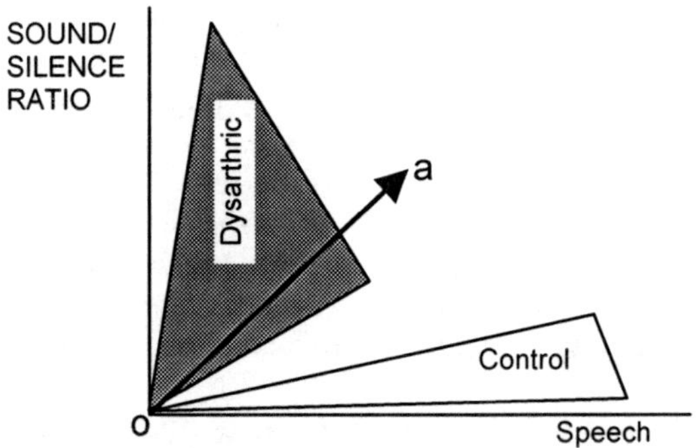

Figure 16.2. Proposed rate/gaps display (Roberts, 2004)

Figure 16.2 shows an example of this measure. A dynamic vector is implemented, with the horizontal axis corresponding to the speech rate parameter and the vertical axis to the ratio of speech:silence (to represent a measure of gaps). The vector, line *o-a* on Figure 16.2, is recalculated at a predefined frequency so that its length, position and variability gives dynamic information to the observer (Roberts, 2004).

To demonstrate the use of this measure, consider a long and stable line running close to the vertical. This would indicate a small proportion of gaps and little change in a slow speech rate. This is shown in Figure 16.2 as the lined region, and is typical of dysarthric speech. Conversely a long or varying length line running close to the horizontal would indicate a significant proportion of gaps with a rate that was high or varying, respectively. This is shown in Figure 16.2 as the dotted region, and is typical of normal speech

The results observed were that all the normal speakers produced vectors which kept near horizontal, with the variability being primarily in rate between individuals depicted by variation in length. Most dysarthric speakers showed a higher degree of scatter but with reduced rate range; the vector angle will change, but the vector has constant length (Simm *et al.,* 2005).

Where speech data are available over a period of months, and there was a detectable change in speech characteristics, the trend is also visible on the vector data (Roberts, 2004). This has the potential for the assessment of improvement, deterioration and fatigue in speech.

16.2.4.2 3-D Cumulative Formant Plots

Prototype software has also been produced to plot novel, real-time, cumulative three-dimensional scatter plots of the lowest formant F1 against the next higher formant F2. The premise of this measure is that the physical influences caused by dysarthric conditions will have specific effects on the formant frequencies that introduce differences from those of normal speech (Simm *et al.,* 2005).

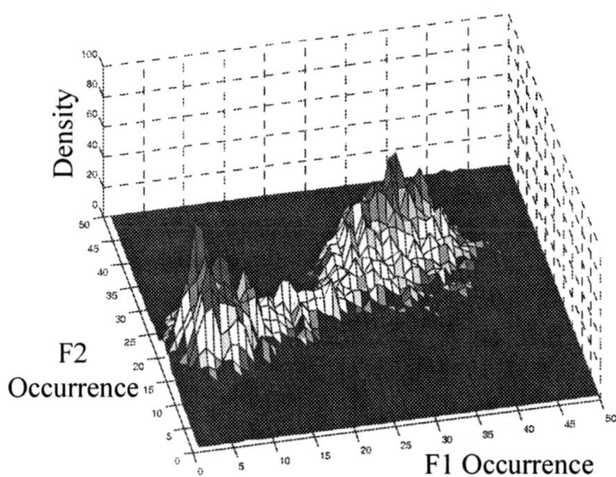

Figure 16.3. 3-D cumulative formant plot showing bipolar distribution (Simm *et al.*, 2005a)

A common method of interpreting the formant frequency data, obtained by spectral analysis, is to plot the amplitude of the lowest frequency formant F1 against that of the next higher formant F2. This is used traditionally for specific sounds, *e.g.* vowels; here the same technique is used over much longer speech samples. This allows the comparison of data collected from people with dysarthria caused by different conditions, and the identification of trends within the data (Simm *et al.,* 2005).

Plotted in this way it is clear to see the three categories of patterns produced as suggested by Roberts (2004). Figure 16.3 shows an example of a bipolar distribution, obtained from moderate to severe dysarthric speech. Samples of normal speech and those of mild dysarthria produce plots with a more evenly scattered data set, with no significant clusters (Simm *et al.,* 2005). Differences in plots can be identified in samples produced from people with different conditions. The deterioration in a person's speech quality can be tracked by comparing differences in the data plots.

16.3 Word Closure

16.3.1 Background

The difference between the way a dysarthric speaker and a normal speaker close a word can be significant as can be seen from Figure 16.4 and Figure 16.5. The waveform in Figure 16.4 shows a typical normal speaker speaking the word "Well" in the context of the following passage:

> *'You wish to know all about my grandfather. Well, he is nearly 90 years old. Yet he still thinks as swiftly as ever.'*

Comparing the normal speech in Figure 16.4 and the moderate-severe dysarthric speech in Figure 16.5, it can be clearly seen and heard that the dysarthric speaker holds onto the "ell" sound in the word much longer than the normal speaker (Simm *et al.*, 2005). The speaker in Figure 16.5 is diagnosed with cerebral palsy.

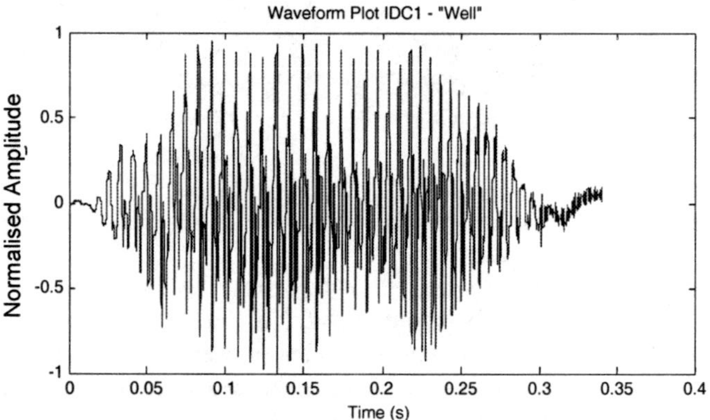

Figure 16.4. Waveform plot of normal speaker – "Well" (Simm *et al.*, 2005b) © IEE 2005

It has been proposed by Simm *et al.* (2005) that these differences are a result of reduced control or an in-coordination in control of the vocal chords and the glottis. This lack of co-ordination or control leads to the speaker being unable to close the glottis appropriately and hence end the voiced "ell" sound effectively.

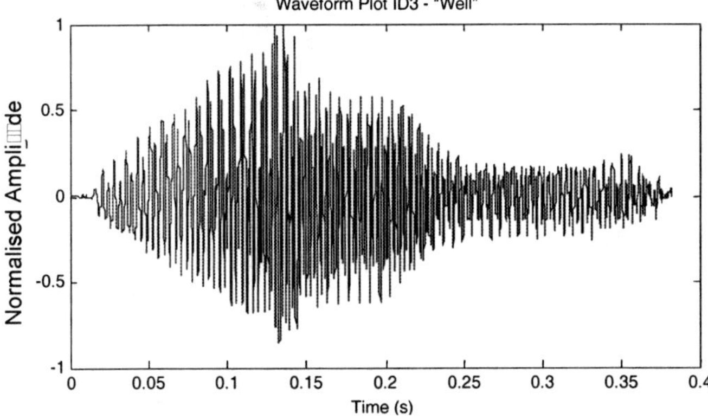

Figure 16.5. Waveform plot of dysarthric speaker "Well" (Cerebral Palsy) (Simm *et al.*, 2005b) © IEE 2005

Figures 16.6 to 16.8 show similar plots to Figure 16.5 for dysarthric speakers with different conditions. The plot in Figure 16.6 is from a stroke-induced dysarthria. This dysarthria was not as severe as in Figure 16.5 and the waveform can be seen to close more abruptly than Figure 16.5, but not so well as the normal speech on a quantitative basis.

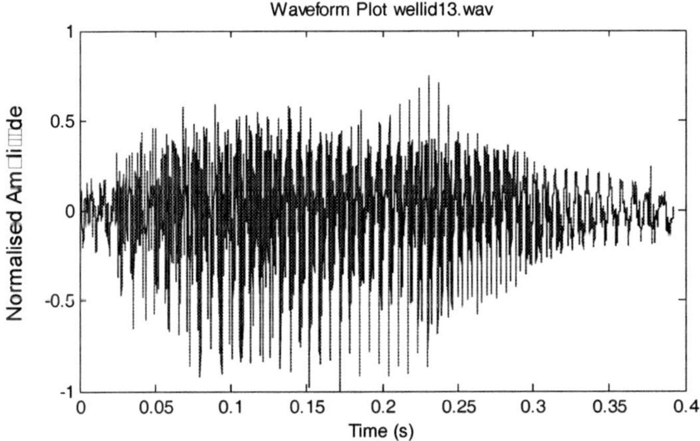

Figure 16.6. Waveform plot of dysarthric speaker "Well" (Stroke)

The speech in Figure 16.7 and 16.8 shows similar characteristics to the other dysarthric samples. The sample in Figure 16.7 was acquired from a moderate dysarthric speaker with cerebella ataxia, and the sample in Figure 16.8 from a mild dysarthric speaker diagnosed with Kennedy's syndrome.

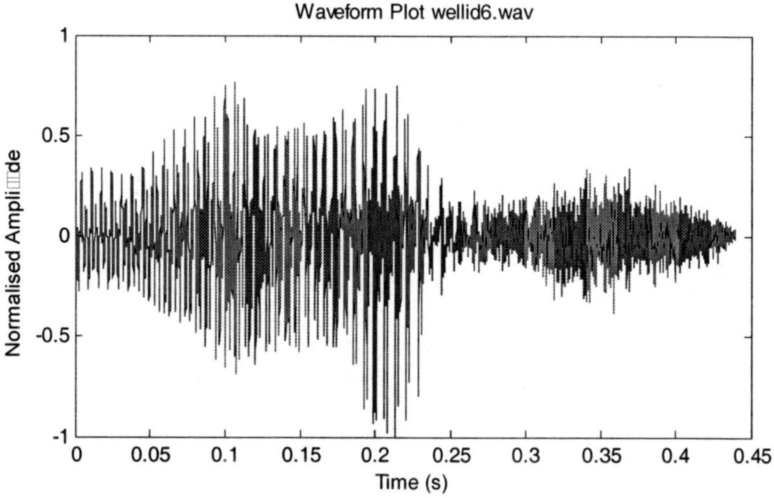

Figure 16.7. Waveform plot of dysarthric speaker "Well" (cerebella ataxia)

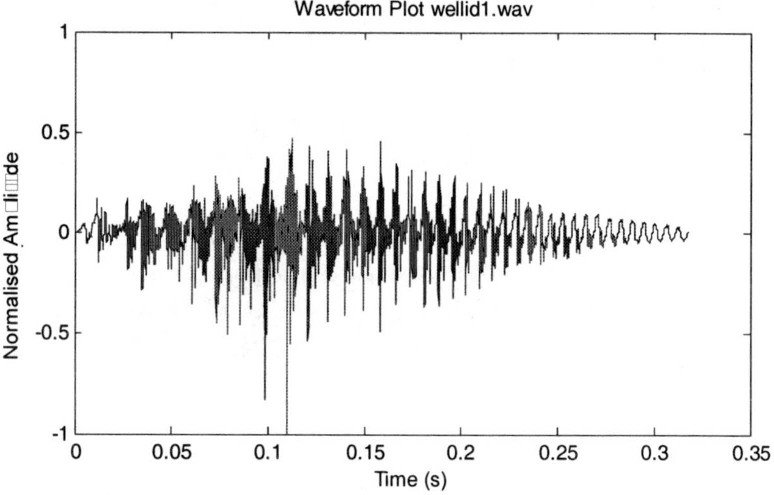

Figure 16.8. Waveform plot of dysarthric speaker "Well" (Kennedy syndrome)

16.3.2 Proposed Closure Metric

A metric designed to assess the degree of control a speaker has of the organs involved in speech production, especially the glottis, would be very useful. Since control of the glottis is linked with swallowing difficulties (dysphagia) (Parse and Kikai, 2004), early diagnosis and therapy could make a large difference to a person's later quality of life.

The measure envisaged entails a software application into which a set passage is spoken, involving words which exercise the closure function of the glottis. This would allow the assessment of the amount of control present, and represent the level of dysarthria. It is proposed that the analysis is done by timing the closure portion of the word as a proportion of the whole spoken word. For instance, in the example used in Figure 16.4 and Figure 16.5, the word "Well", the ratio of the time taken to say "ll" after the detectable vowel sound "e" as a proportion of the whole word would give an indication as to the length of the closure. An average "closure time" for certain words in the passage would produce the assessment. This analysis could be undertaken automatically by detecting the end of the characteristic vowel sound and timing to the end of the word.

16.4 Conclusions

The two prototypes discussed have already received favourable reactions from SLT professionals (Simm *et al.*, 2005). The rate/gaps display with the angular component and varying length vector gives near real-time feedback to the observer which may help the speaker pace his/her speech delivery (Roberts, 2004). The 3D cumulative formant plots demonstrate correspondence with changes in dysarthria over time and may also aid diagnosis of condition (Simm *et al.*, 2005).

The current research into the analysis of the word closure characteristics of speech may lead to further insight into the assessment of dysarthric speech and may have implications for the diagnosis of other disorders such as dysphagia. The word closure work has been furthered here to include these areas.

If the closure metric proves valuable to SLTs, then along with the rate/gaps display and 3-D formant plots it can be developed into a suite of software tools. The suite would be designed to aid the diagnosis of dysarthria-causing conditions and track changes in speech quality. Through consultation with SLTs it is clear this type of software would be very useful to both health care professionals and people with speech impairments.

16.5 Acknowledgements

Thanks go to Claire Philpott of the Morecambe Bay NHS Primary Care Trust for her assistance in selecting subjects for speech data collection, assisting collection sessions, and acting as a consultant to the research. This research is funded by the Engineering and Physical Sciences Research Council.

16.6 References

Harel BT, Cannizzaro MS, Cohen H, Reilly N, Snyder PJ (2004) Acoustic characteristics of Parkinsonian speech: a potential biomarker of early disease progression and treatment. Journal of Neurolinguistics 17: 439–453

Laver J (1994) Principles of phonetics. Cambridge University Press, UK

Lemmetty S (1999) Review of speech synthesis technology. Available at: http://www.acoustics.hut.fi/~slemmett/dippa/

Love R, Webb W (1992) Neurology for the speech-language pathologist, 2nd edn. Butterworth-Heinemann, Oxford, UK

Max L, Mueller PB (1996) Speaking F_0 and cepstral periodicity analysis of conversational speech in a 105-year-old woman: variability of ageing effects. Journal of Voice 10: 245–251

NIDCD (2004) National Institute on Deafness and other communication disorders glossary. Available at: http://www.nidcd.nih.gov/health/glossary/glossary.asp

Prasse JW, Kikano GE (2004) An overview of dysphagia in the elderly. Advanced Studies in Medicine 4(10): 527–533

Roberts PE (2004) Improvement of computer recognition and development of new metrics. PhD-thesis, Lancaster University, UK

Simm WA, Roberts PE, Joyce MJ, Philpott C (2005a) The quantitative assessment of dysarthric speech for rse in evidence-based speech therapy. In: Proceedings of HCI International 2005, Las Vegas, USA

Simm WA, Roberts PE, Joyce MJ (2005b) Signal processing for use in the assessment of dysarthric speech. In: Proceedings of the 3rd IEE International Seminar on Medical Applications of Signal Processing, London, UK

Chapter 17

Non-formal Therapy and Learning Potentials Through Human Gesture Synchronised to Robotic Gesture

E. Petersson and A. Brooks

17.1 Introduction

This paper reports a non-formal therapeutic approach where severely disabled children were encouraged to "play" utilising whatever physical ability they had. Human gesture was thus empowered to control synchronous robotic movement and multimedia feedback within an interactive Virtual Environment (VE) where the participant was free of functional expectations and consequences.

The study is contained within a larger body of research titled SoundScapes which is based on stimulation of the human through interactive experiences using non-intrusive interfaces. The research has been appraised as giving potential in human afferent efferent neural loop closure (often called sensory-motor or stimuli-response chain; Scherer, 2000), Figure 17.1.

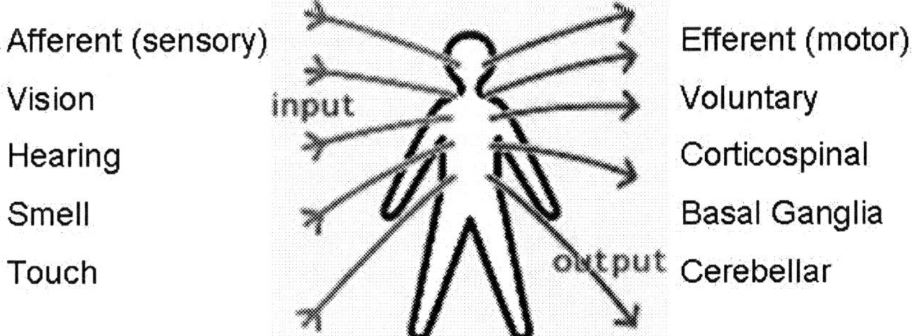

Figure 17.1. Human afferent-efferent neural loop closure

Intervention strategies should not detract from the therapy or interfere with the patient's well-being. These should be motivational and inspiring for both therapist and user and promote non-verbal interactions. Thus, this approach considers non-formal therapy as unintended therapy that encourages an immersed play mindset in the therapy session. As such the approach offers a resource for fun and expressive interaction. Thereby, non-formal therapy always has a character that motivates the individual and is motivated by an interest to find the best possible form for expression. Accordingly, when working with severely disabled children idiosyncratic attributes must be addressed so as to take account of variation in facility, preferences and limitations. An ability in the therapist to improvise and optimise the situation within the 'patient-therapist' sessions is expected and this is optimised through knowledge of the tools and the subject. In this way conditions encouraging creativity become central to the potential for learning and the optimisation of the situation.

The aim of this paper was to explore learning potentials through interactive play situations. The objective of the study was to create a virtual coach as a supplement for the therapist where a 'wireless' links between human and robot enabled control without encumbrance from attachments and wires.

17.2 Background

In the last decade robotic devices have been created specifically for human interaction so as to motivate subsequent behaviour (Shibata, 1997). These devices have been used in children's wards and elderly wards in hospitals as well as at senior citizens' homes in 'robot-therapy' sessions. Robot therapy is not new. Hogan (2000) details the training of an arm of a person disabled by a stroke which is interacting with a device resembling a robotic arm able to measure the force being exerted by the user. Related work in rehabilitation robotics (Cook *et al.*, 2002) showed that the development of a robot manipulator could facilitate learning by young children who were generally unable to grasp objects or speak.

We began working with non-intrusive sensor gesture control of motorised light devices in 1994. This was with the originating human movement being captured by first generation SoundScapes infrared sensors and mapped for device control.

Each channel was mapped to control the light [channel 1 = pan] [channel 2 = tilt] [channel 3 = Z] where Z was selectable between light pattern, colour, or speed. The control was to a motorised mirror assembly on the device that was most often located at a distance from the participant empowered to control. This movement data that empowered manipulation of light change was also mapped to sound patches on a digital synthesiser or sampler. The closure of the afferent-efferent neural loop, Figure 17.1, is reinforced through this strategy. A decade later, developments led to physical-to-physical control by children who had severe motor retardation through the moving head interaction.

17.2.1 Interactive Play

For a child with severe disabilities play situations can be more or less impossible and accompanied by frustration for the child due to limited access to suitable tools for expression. Consequently, this affects the learning and fun potential for the child. Most play research describes its relationship to children's cognitive development, and focuses on solitary play (Rogoff, 1990). However, this research does not account for the totality of what is going on in situations of interactive play. Our approach to play is activity driven and based on Aesthetic Resonance (Brooks and Hasselblad, 2004; Brooks and Petersson, 2005c), which is to say an immersed engagement where the interaction makes the child forget the physical movement involved in the conveying of his or her intention.

In related work play in the form of intrinsic motivated exploration is considered as an important resource for non-formal learning (Petersson, 2000; Aderklou *et al.*, 2001; Bigün *et al.*, 2003; Petersson, 2004). This is similar to what Csikszentmihalyi (1992) names as autotelic activity, which is characterised as being carried out for its own sake with inner goals generating the state of flow. The robotic system used in play may be viewed as a support for the child to reach beyond his or her current level of development (Vygotsky, 1978). An adjusted support for the child is offered by the interaction with the robotic system, which challenges the child to reach a level of mastery. Rogoff (1990) names the process of support "transfer of responsibility" (p. 201). Inherent is the balance between challenge and sensibility that allows and encourages change. This, in turn, can result in an experience of self-agency and gained competence. In the terms used by Vygotsky (1987) this is characterised by two simultaneous processes; on the one hand it concerns use of technical tools and on the other hand it concerns mediation of psychological tools. Hence, in our approach there is a constant transformation of existing interactions and the constant making of new interactions in an on-going process between the robotic device, the child, and the facilitator, all guided by the child's and the facilitator's individual interest. Thereby, the child's perception of the social world as well as the affective state emerges into new interactions as expressions of the child's interest. This is the process which we describe as learning.

17.2.2 Design and Creativity

Interacting with robotics includes specifics to interaction, which, iteratively, become part of the responsive robotic system. Inclusive participation by the facilitator is inherent in designing the interactive responsive environment where the interaction with the robotic system takes place. Related work emphasises the facilitator's role in participatory and recursive analysis of data (Brooks and Petersson, 2005a). Accordingly, the inclusive participation optimises a mutual understanding of the child's engagement with the robotic system. By this, the facilitator can reflect *in* action and, afterwards, *on* actions. This then raises the question of the facilitator's selective decisions about which mode to use in order to optimise the interactive play situation.

This cycle of reflections constitutes a creative design approach as it can be used as a means to empower children's communication, play, and expression. Consequently, through inclusive participation the child also has a share as a directly and indirectly involved partner in the creative design of its own interactive responsive play environment. Related studies (Petersson and Bengtsson, 2004) emphasise that a facilitator's trust in the abilities of 'participants' in a process like this increases their sense of participation in the situation. In the case of children with severe disabilities creative design decisions and planning of the play situations are the key to success. Thus, creativity is an important element of the interaction between the child and the facilitator. We suggest that it is through inclusive participation that the facilitator makes a significant impact, by manually optimising the therapy situation. Through this, the child and the facilitator develop means for an inter-subjective and joyful learning experience, which supports the child's creative achievements. Optimally, this results in a masterful performance encouraging explorations without immediate goals as in play (Berg, 1992), which are characteristic of a non-formal approach to therapy rather than traditional forms (Brooks and Petersson, 2005b; Brooks and Petersson, 2005c).

Behaviours indicating play sequences are in our case based on gestures of the user where a deliberate exploration of the 'interactive information space' is subject to transformational sequences throughout which the user is able to detect the causality of his/her affecting interaction with the robotic device. Fagan (1981) suggests that 'using a tool' is an example of such effects. We focus upon the use of an interactive robotic device as the "tool" for the therapist to utilise as a virtual coach to help produce beneficial effects.

17.3 Method

The method used was (1) observation of interaction between children with severe disabilities and responsive 'synchronous to gesture in real-time' robotic devices functioning as a virtual coach, to determine learning potentials, and (2) a questionnaire to facilitators. In this way it may be possible to define characteristics of a robotic virtual coach for use in rehabilitation and habilitation, as a supplement to traditional therapy.

Such characteristics are suggested as a layered approach which has at the top most level a user-perceived interactive "play" environment. The interaction was tailored to each individual. Inclusive participation and a creative design approach, see Section 17.2.2, were elements of the methodology.

17.3.1 Subjects

The institutes involved were asked to volunteer children who were all able to see and hear. The children were from the community that is classified in Scandinavia as Profound Multi Learning Disabled (PMLD). At all sessions there was a knowledgeable carer to ensure no discomfort for the child. Four children between 4 and 6 years of age were selected in collaboration with the institute.

17.3.2 Equipment

An eight channel moving light controller (Elektralite CP10) capable of translation of MIDI to DMX 512 was central to the system. The robotic device chosen was the moving head MiniMAC Profile intelligent lighting unit that projects multi-colour light patterns of high contrast at up to 540 degrees of pan and up to 270 degrees of tilt. Three MiniMAC Profile moving head units were used. The Cycling74 software Max was used for mapping.

17.3.3 Session Procedure

A basic child assessment coding scale for each session was established by asking the carer (1) how the child was perceived at the start of every session, (2) how the child was perceived during the session, and (3) how the child was perceived following the return to the institute. Sensor selection and set up was logged to a user profile. The set up of the sessions was in a large empty room so that the full range of the robotic moving heads could be programmed to extend beyond the user's peripheral field of view so that a head movement was required to observe at full extremities.

As shown in Figure 17.2, the user was positioned near the centre of the room with a camera behind to capture the scene. A second camera was positioned in front to capture facial expression. A sensor was set up according to the user's capability of movement. Infrared volumetric sensors and ultrasound were used.

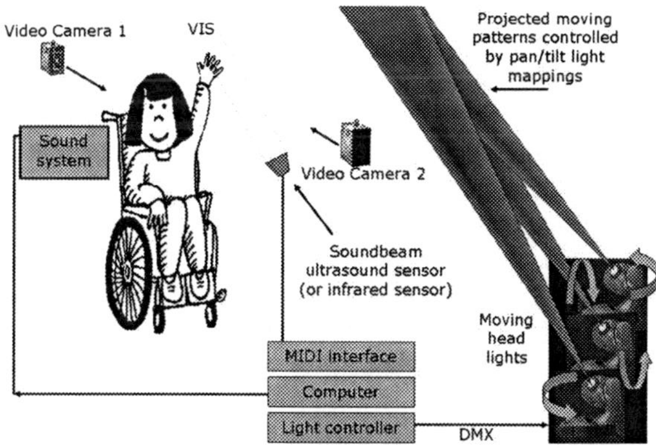

Figure 17.2. Set up: human gesture captured by sensor mapped to devices

17.3.4 Analysis Method

Video annotation was central to the analysis. The coding system was individual to each child and created with assistance from the carer who was familiar with the child's various responses. As best as possible we generalised common expressions among the children accounting for each child having individual faculty limitations and abilities. Typical features such as a smile, a mouth opening, a quieting, an eye focus, a frown, hand or lower torso movement were noted. Our parallel research with children in virtual environments (Brooks and Petersson, 2005b) used a camera based software algorithm to analyse quantity and segmentation of movement and pauses. However due to the dynamic light change in the dark room and the use of infrared night vision hardware causing unexpected reflected IR back to the sensors this could not be used, as spurious readings were evident.

17.4 Results

The results are based on the analysis of three "robotic light interaction" sessions with each of the four children involved in the study and the analysis of questionnaires answered by four carers. The child's facial expressions and torso movements were the basic unit of analysis. Our findings reported that it was useful to apply an inclusive participative analysis of the video material to understand critical emerging elements in the children's actions and interactions.

The results pointed to learning potentials from Human Robotic Interaction (HRI) within a Virtual Environment (VE). The choice of the MiniMac profile robotic intelligent light devices was astute. The units responded with a latency of around half a second which was acceptable but not optimal. We tested various gobos (patterns) and colours but could not ascertain if they were making a difference to the child.

17.4.1 Observations

Most of the sessions lasted around 30 minutes, with the shortest at 11 minutes and the longest at 46 minutes. Each session timeline involved dynamic interaction and response showing a recurring pattern. One child was not comfortable in his chair so we adapted his position by placing him on a floor mat that was adjusted so that he was able to see the light patterns. One child was asleep when entering the Virtual Interactive Space (VIS) in one session. Slowly he woke and explored with playful head movements that controlled the device, simultaneously with the projected light patterns and sounds.

The ratio and sensitivity of gesture to resulting feedback were totally programmable and limited only by the physical constraints of the hardware and room location.

The four children showed immersion in every session through an observed consciousness of intent. The twelve-picture sheet in the Figure 17.3 illustrates moments from the sessions where immersion was apparent. These pictures alone cannot tell the whole story, but only hint at the explorations and experiences gained.

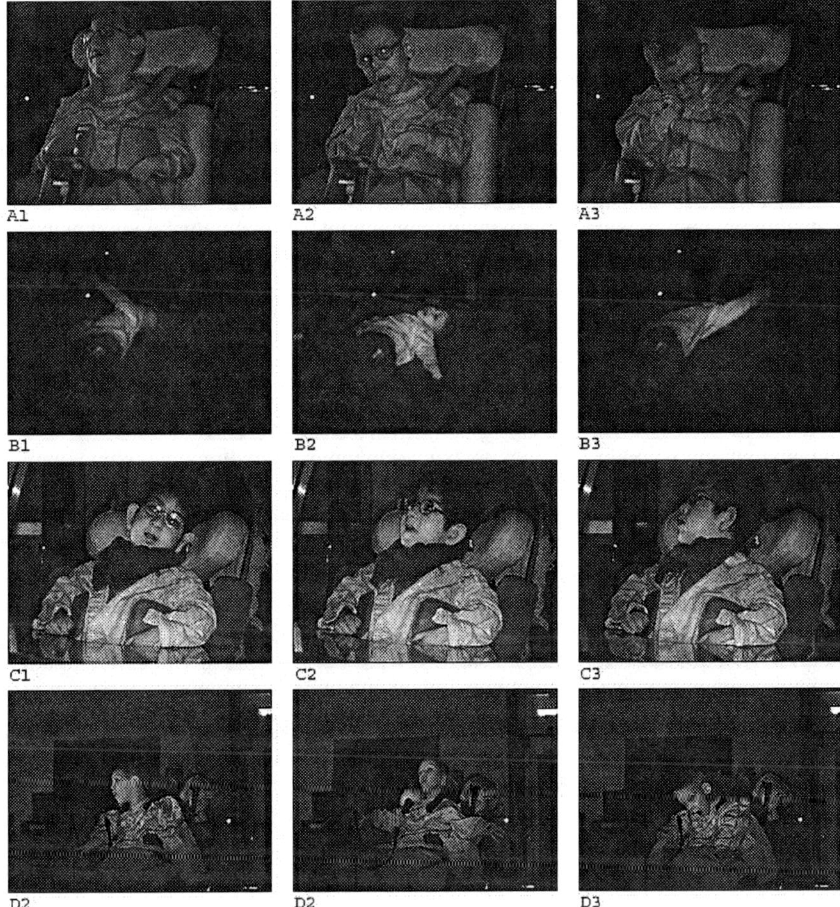

Figure 17.3. Immersed interaction with robotic device via head and hand gesticulation. The quality of the images is low because a night vision setting with the camera was used.

One child was immersed in dynamic explorations of what was happening under his control and explored the interactive space further through varying the range, the speed and direction of his gesture – he indicated awareness of a direct correspondence with and control of the physical movement of the robot head and the subsequent movement of the lights. Such self-achievement is a rare commodity for such children.

The facial expressions of one child when he was exploring the virtual interactive space pointed towards awareness and enjoyment as he was empowered to manipulate the robotic device. The physical relationship of synchronised child movement to robot movement reinforced the activity of the child.

The sessions followed a recurring pattern similar to that in children's play, where as exploration gives way to play the emphasis changes from the question of "what does this object do?" to "what can I do with this object?" The study showed that the sequence was extended along similar lines with further emphasis changes: "when I move - the light patterns move:" "when I move - I hear sounds:"..." when I stop moving I neither hear sounds nor see the light patterns moving!" ... "Hey I'm in control here- and it's fun!" And further one might suggest that the emphasis was extended to "well nobody told me what I should do, or for how long, so I will just have more fun with what I have learnt I can do with this object!" In the sessions all children continued to explore until they indicated, through reduced engagement, that it was time to stop. This was observed through the face monitor by the child's carer who was watching the monitor which showed images from the front camera at all times throughout the sessions.

17.4.2 Questionnaires

The comments on the series of sessions given by each child's carer were positive. The carers stated that the children were tired following the return to the institute after the sessions and that the physical exercise of whatever limited abilities they had was a positive way to energise their available skills. The children were generally observed to be more content and happier after the session. Following the end of the series of sessions, the children were seen to be aware of social contact at a slightly higher level, and three of the four showed indications of improved eye to hand co-ordination and concentration.

On subsequent contact with the institute approximately one month after the end of the sessions, the carers stated that the children showed no significant long term improvement compared to their condition prior to the limited numbers of sessions. The initial elevated happiness had returned to the same level as before the study.

17.5 Discussion and Conclusions

Reflecting on the sessions, the set-ups could have been improved, especially the sensor location for gesture capture from the human user. The sensor should be remotely controlled from a distance so as not to interfere with the user and should also be wireless. This has been addressed in the latest generation of sensors.

Front camera night vision infrared needs to be tested to see if impingement on the subject corrupts the received data at sensor. This is because of the spurious readings mentioned in the text.

Through interactive play in virtual environments a child could acquire new abilities, interactions, expressions and emotions, enabling a mastering of tasks and practising of skills. As such, the interactive play situations indicated an enhancement of the quality of play and learning, which, in turn, facilitated immersive explorations that were utilised in the therapy. This is to say that play had a motivational potential resulting from the interactive virtual environment. The children's concentration when interacting with the robotic system furthermore emphasised the autotelic quality of the play.

The virtual interactive environment had the potential to evoke the child's interest in practising otherwise limited skills. Rogoff (1990) underlines that interest has a motivating character that channels the child's choices of actions. Through practising skills the child experienced a sense of control and, thereby, mastery of the therapy situation. So we would like to suggest that interest influences the child's development of competencies and related self-esteem in a positive way. The main point we would like to make here is that these aspects show that non-formal therapy is an opportunity to expand the child's learning experiences, as learning is so closely related to play and intrinsic motivation.

Our assessment of the contented happiness factor is that it may have come from empowered activity resulting in the achievement of control by the child, whereby the success factor, often unattainable by children with such severe disabilities, was contributing to their emotional self-esteem.

The inclusive participation approach was a fruitful base for creative design to be further investigated in future studies. The approach was rich in promoting collaboration on different levels of participation: on child and facilitator level, and on researcher and facilitator level. Overall, the collaboration motivated the participants to achieve more than they would have been able to individually. Hence, we would like to suggest that inclusive participation has the potential to support the emergence of new and improved forms of actions and interactions, in the design of therapy as well as in the design of research.

This study underlines the importance of inclusive participation, which is to say the necessity of collaboration between the child, the facilitator and the researchers to optimise the interaction with the robotic system. Based on this system, the character of the virtual coach is dependent on the physical coach, the facilitator, guidancing by manual intervention so as to maintain an optimisation of the child's state of flow in actions and interactions. The latter is inherent with creative design to empower interactive play experiences in therapy sessions.

In conclusion, further studies are needed to define the character of a virtual coach. However, based on the results indicated from this study we suggest that the virtual coach should be motivating the designer of the robotic system so as to:

- be non-invasive;
- have a "silent" space available, *i.e.* no interaction;
- be intuitive, *i.e.* offer a direct contact with the content feedback.

Finally, more research, especially based on inclusive, participatory, and creative design methods, is needed to study the potential of using robotics for children with severe disabilities, as well as to develop models of application. Furthermore, we emphasise the need to develop appropriate techniques, means of measurements, and instruments that are suitable to assess results and impact of the research.

17.6 Acknowledgements

The authors wish to thank the institute staff and children involved in the study as well as Center for Advanced Visualization and Interactivity (CAVI), Aarhus, Denmark where the research was hosted.

17.7 References

Aderklou C, Fritzdorf L, Petersson E (2001) Pl@yground: pedagogical innovation and play products created to expand self-development through child collaboration through computer-mediated-communication (CMC). Socrates, Leonardo and Youth, Halmstad University, Sweden

Berg L-E (1992) The playing human (in Swedish). Studentlitteratur, Lund University, Sweden

Bigün J, Petersson E, Dahiya R (2003) Multimodal interfaces – designing digital artefacts together with children. In: Proceedings of the 7th International Conference on Learning and Educational Media, Bratislava, Slovakia

Brooks A, Hasselblad S (2004) CAREHERE – creating aesthetically resonant environments for the handicapped, elderly and rehabilitation: Sweden. In: Proceedings of ICDVRAT 2004, Oxford, UK

Brooks A, Petersson E (2005a) Recursive reflection and learning in raw data video analysis of interactive 'play' environments for special needs health care. In: Proceedings of Healthcom2005, Busan, Korea

Brooks A, Petersson E (2005b) Raw emotional signalling, via expressive behavior. In: Proceedings of the 15th International Conference on Artificial Reality and Telexistence, University of Canterbury, Christchurch, New Zealand (in press)

Brooks A, Petersson E (2005c) Play therapy utilizing Sony EyeToy®. In: Proceedings or the 8th International Workshop on Presence, University College of London, UK

Cook AM, Meng MQH, Gu JJ, Howery K (2002) Development of a robotic device for facilitating learning by children who have severe disabilities. IEEE Transactions on Neural and Rehabilitation Engineering 10(3): 178–187

Csikszentmihalyi M (1992) Flow: the psychology of optimal experience. Natur och Kultur

Fagan R (1981) Animal play behavior. Oxford University Press, New York, USA

Hogan N (2000) MIT-Manus robot aids physical therapy of stroke victims. MIT, Boston, USA

Petersson E (2000) Innovative play products – development of toys for children's play and rehabilitation. In: Proceedings of the SNAFA, Halmstad University, Sweden

Petersson E (2004) Using and developing new learning technologies by integrating physical and virtual toy systems. Socrates, Leonardo & Youth, Halmstad University, Halmstad, Sweden

Petersson E, Bengtsson J (eds.) (2004) Encouraging co-operation as participation – the beginning of a beautiful friendship? European Commission, Innovation Program, Transfer of Innovative Methods. Halmstad University, Halmstad, Sweden

Rogoff B (1990) Apprenticeship in thinking. Cognitive development in social context. Oxford University Press, New York, USA

Scherer K (2000) Emotion. In: Hewstone M, Stoebe W (eds.), 3rd edn. Introduction to social psychology: a European perspective. Blackwell, Oxford, UK

Shibata T, Irie R (1997) Artificial emotional creature for human-robot interaction – a new direction for intelligent system. In: Proceedings of the IEEE/ASME International Conference on Advanced Intelligent Mechatronics, Alberque, New Mexico, USA

Vygotsky LS (1978) Mind in society. Harvard University, Cambridge, USA

Vygotsky LS (1987) The collected works of L. S. Vygotsky. Vol. 1. Problems of general psychology. Plenum, New York, USA

Part IV

Understanding Users and Involving Them in the Design Process

Chapter 18

Inclusive Design Evaluation and the Capability-demand Relationship

U. Persad, P.M. Langdon and P.J. Clarkson

18.1 Introduction

In the product design process, designers require systematic methods, tools and data in support of product design evaluation (Clarkson and Keates, 2003). The accessibility of everyday products such as toasters, telephones, microwave cookers, remote controls, and numerous other products, is an important attribute of product quality. Understanding the accessibility of a product requires understanding the interaction relationship between the artefact's features and users' capabilities. Thus, there is a need to measure or estimate the level of accessibility for any given product to ensure that is satisfies the largest number of people.

This paper addresses the problem of supporting product evaluation in inclusive design by analysis of the interaction of user capabilities with properties of product interfaces. The goal is to map the necessary user capability data to product designs in the form of measurement scales that can be used in product audits to estimate design exclusion. As such, this approach is a form of user-centred design that extends the approaches of usability, human factors engineering, ergonomics and interaction design (Stanton, 1998) to the wider population with various disabilities.

18.1.1 Product Design Evaluation

Hartson describes two ways in which an evaluation can be conducted – analytical and empirical (Hartson *et al.*, 2001). Analytical methods are based on an analysis of product features and characteristics while empirical evaluation investigates product design performance when it is placed in actual usage situations. These two categories also reflect the level of user participation in the evaluation process. Analytical-intrinsic methods use collected data on various user characteristics and expert opinion while empirical-payoff methods require actual user involvement in user trials and observations. For our purpose, we consider developing support for analytical, inspection based evaluation methods by utilising scales of user capability. In addition, properties of activities and tasks in the use of the product are also considered.

18.1.2 Previous Capability Scales

Recent research into inclusive design (Keates and Clarkson, 2002) has investigated the relationship between capabilities of the population at large and guidelines for the design of features of products. This research suggests that a good representation of the capability range of individuals can be made on a three-axis scale derived from the basic psychological dimensions of sensory, motor and cognitive capability. This work builds on previous work on using capability scales to assess the demands made on users by product features (Keates and Clarkson, 2003).

There are many sources of capability data, one such being the Older Adultdata (Smith *et al.,* 1998). However, recent research has focused on one of the most complete representative disability data sets; the 1996/97 Great Britain Disability Follow-up Survey (DFS). This survey was based on a measure of severity of disability established through the consensus of judges including medical experts and disabled people (Martin and Elliot, 1992; Semmence, 1998). The DFS survey introduced thirteen capability scales of which seven are most relevant to product evaluation: locomotion, dexterity, reach and stretch, vision, hearing, communication, and intellectual functioning.

Though these scales were found to have advantages such as coherence, utility, and statistical validity, they also presented certain disadvantages: (1) They do not represent the discontinuous, non-linear nature of capability loss; (2) The scale points do not map directly to product interfaces; (3) Multiple impairments are dealt with using a naive linear additive model; (4) Some scales confound a number of underlying capabilities. In addition, the scales were founded on judges' notions of disability and a self-report questionnaire rather than objective measurement (Dong *et al.,* 2002; Langdon *et al.,* 2003).

18.1.3 Development of New Scales

In order to address these shortcomings of the capability scales and to underpin the application of such scales to an analytical evaluation process, we propose the following simple framework shown in Figure 18.1.

Inclusive design requires an understanding of the user capability and product demand relationship. As Figure 18.1 shows, a product interface consists of various entities (such as text, buttons, dials, connectors, LCD displays *etc.*) with various attributes such as material, colour, shape, force characteristics, and dimensions. The values of these attributes in a particular product design determine the demands that the product makes on the user. For example, a product's visual demand is set by the choice of size, colour and contrast of text on the product. In turn, a user must have the ability to see and read the text in order for it to be accessible.

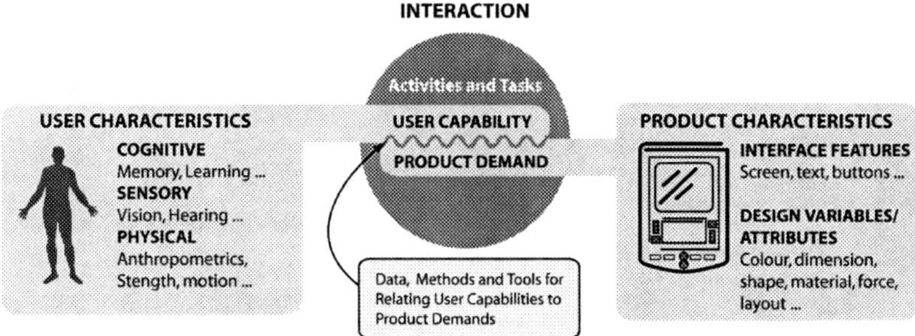

Figure 18.1. A simple illustration of the relationship between user sensory, cognitive and physical capabilities and the demands made on the user by the product

18.1.4 Evaluation System Requirements

The requirements of the evaluation system are: (1) that its output is in a form that is easily comprehended by the designer irrespective of the complexity of the user-product interaction and (2) that it should be sensitive to variations in product features that can lead to sensory, physical and cognitive exclusion. In addition, (3) it should be applicable to everyday products without onerous computation or knowledge searches and (4) it should be implemented in such a way that it is possible to estimate the changes in excluded population that occur with specific design changes.

When a user uses any given product, design exclusion takes place when the demands of certain interface features exceed the user's capabilities. If, for example, a user does not possess the required visual acuity, contrast sensitivity and colour perception to detect a text label, then design exclusion takes place. This can be remedied by adjusting the product attributes (the text size, font, colour and background colour) to reduce the capability demand. In this way, by systematically minimising the capability demands of a given product interface, a more accessible product can be designed.

Evaluation scales can aid in this process of mapping the demand profile of the product to the capability profiles of users. By using the notion of scales of variation in human capability, a designer can see how various interface components comparatively map to these capability distributions and what changes need to be made to the design variables in order to reduce the capability demands. Figure 18.2 shows a schematic overview of an evaluation framework that maps sensory, physical and cognitive demands of products to capability distributions in order to estimate design exclusion.

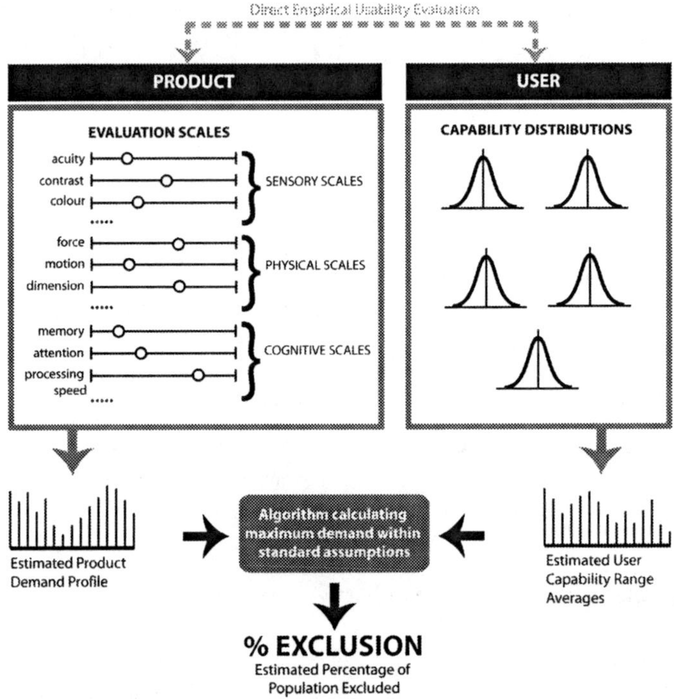

Figure 18.2. Overview of a framework to estimate design exclusion

Empirical approaches to evaluation have been successful in evaluating specific interfaces (Keates and Clarkson, 2004). However, these methods can be laborious, time-consuming and prone to sample bias. They are also constrained to interface-capability interactions that only reveal themselves during usability trials. Hence these approaches are limited by the interactions of the specific users recruited to participate. Drawing conclusions from such trials on accessibility for the wider heterogeneous population of less capable users can be misleading. By using scales of capability demand to assess the product, features that cause design exclusion may be discovered that might not have been picked up in a specific user trial or observational study. Analytical approaches based on measured population data allow for a population perspective that is essential for inclusive design (Persad *et al.*, 2005). It is important to note that we advocate a balance between empirical and analytic approaches, using the advantages of analytical methods to compensate for the disadvantages of empirical methods and vice versa.

A set of capability sub-scales is needed that is based on a breakdown of each of the key perceptual, physical and cognitive dimensions that account for most of the variability in the majority of human interface interaction. Combining these scale results together forms an estimate of the ability demand made by the product as a single profile. This profile is then matched against user capability profiles (population data). Exclusion can be calculated by comparison of product demand and capability ranges for differing age groups and capability limitations. Such a system must deal with capability variation resulting from multiple impairments, as well as the equivalent range of perceptual, physical and cognitive requirements of product features. It is assumed that variation and interactions of this sort can be minimised by the use of normal assumptions. Examples include assuming a general position and orientation of viewing for visual features, the use of single or multiple limbs in physical features and trade-offs of speed against accuracy for cognitive attributes.

However, before such evaluation scales can be developed, certain issues need to be addressed, including what user capabilities need to be considered in sub-scales and how product interfaces should be decomposed in order to construct the demand profile.

18.2 Users Capabilities and Product Interfaces

18.2.1 User Capabilities

User characteristics in the performance of user actions on product interfaces can be broken down into the sensory, cognitive and motor dimensions (Keates and Clarkson, 2002). Though individual human characteristics can be measured (such as strength, grip, visual acuity, short term memory capacity, speed of processing *etc.*), the ways that these basic characteristics combine in the performance of various real world task demands is complex.

One method of dealing with this complexity and predicting human performance based on lower level elemental resources is described by Kondraske in his Elemental Resources Model (Kondraske, 1995). This model uses the mathematics of resource economics and the concept of the limiting basic elements of performance. It is one of a number of extant models that could be used to estimate the level of performance of user actions based on underlying ability. Other models are also being investigated which could deal with imprecision in the measurement of human characteristics.

18.2.2 Product Interface Features

In order to understand better the demands a given product makes on user capabilities, the product interface must first be analysed and classified via a suitable systematic analysis method. Product interfaces expose the functionality of the product via various displays and controls. The properties of the interface thus need to be identified in order to assess their impact on the user's capability level. Table 18.1 shows some product attributes that form user demands.

Table 18.1. Interface attributes that affect product demands

Sensory	*Visual Demand* – sizes/dimensions of features, shape/form of features, material colour, contrast with background, movement, specularity, salience, … *Auditory Demand* – Pitch, amplitude, timbre/harmonics … *Haptic-Tactile Demand* – control resistance and properties, material surface finishing, shape of object, weight and temperature of objects in operation, …
Cognitive	Display/control layout complexity, language and wording, symbols used, memory requirements, speed of use requirements, demanded task sequence, multiple attention demands …
Physical / Motor	Sizes/dimensions of objects, shape/form of objects, material surface finish, operating force characteristics, motion required for operation (linear, rotational or combination), interface layout and size, …

18.2.3 Approach to Classifying the Interface

Our approach to developing a suitable classification scheme for product interfaces involves proposing a scheme and gradually improving it over various iterations of validation with observational data. This is so that weaknesses in the classification can be strengthened as it is checked against empirical data of user-product interaction. The following Table 18.2 summarises this general approach to analysis of the interface. In the first instance, the product interface can be broken down in an object-oriented fashion listing the interface features together with relevant properties (as in Figure 18.4). Then, the sensory, physical and cognitive elements need to be extracted as shown in Table 18.2.

It is important to note that a description of the task sequence has to be considered in addition to a decomposition of the interface features into sensory, cognitive and physical demands. This could be derived from a brief usability task analysis or cognitive walkthrough. This will enable the determination of importance (or weighting values) for different interface features based on the frequency of usage.

Table 18.2. Classifying the product interface

Sensory Displays *e.g.* screens, text, symbols, audio sounds on all interface elements.	Identify all the main sensory displays on the product together with associated properties. Map to sensory capability scales (for vision, hearing and tactile senses). Sensory displays with maximum and minimum demands can be identified.
Physical/Manipulation elements *e.g.* product chassis, control buttons and knobs, connectors	Identify the interface features that require physical interaction and manipulation together with associated properties. Map to physical capability scales (for anthropometric, motion and force capabilities). Elements with maximum and minimum demands can be identified.
Controls Mapping, Feedback and Layout	Identify important controls on the product and determine the demands on user cognition.
Mental Model	Identify the procedural and declarative mental models necessary for using the product, and determine cognitive demands.
Affordances	Identify the various cognitive, sensory and physical affordances and determine how well the product affords these actions to users with lower capability.

Once the demand profile of the product is established, it can be systematically mapped to scales of user capability. Conceptually, this is illustrated in Figure 18.3. If a product interface feature demands a user capability at a certain level (say a visual demand at 1cm text height, Arial font, green colour on a white background), an estimate is required of the overall visual demand on that feature. Users with visual capability lower than this level (*i.e.* they do not have the acuity, contrast sensitivity and colour perception to detect the text) will be excluded.

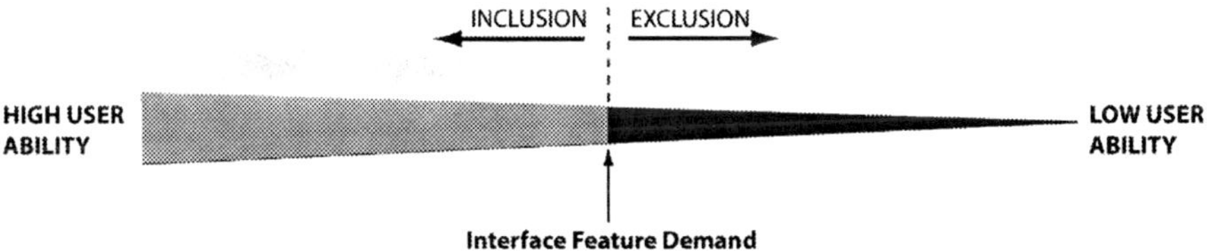

Figure 18.3. The mapping of an interface demand to a scale of capability

18.3 Observational Study

In order to better understand the capability-demand relationship, a pilot analytic observational study was conducted with a simple toaster (Figure 18.4). Examples from this study will be used to illustrate the analysis of the product interface demands.

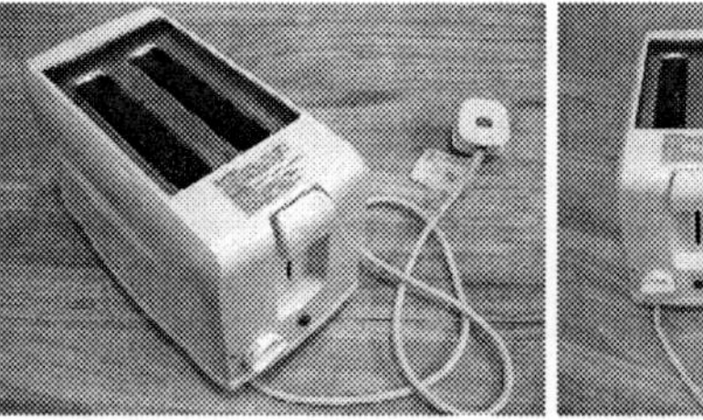

Figure 18.4. Simple toaster used in the study with the following interface properties: 1) Toaster Body/Chassis, 2) Two Slots for bread slices, 3) Slider Handle, 4) STOP button, 5) Toasting rotating heating control (with text), 6) Plug and cord, 7) Crumb Removal Tray, 8) Instructions/Warning label and 9) Brand name text label

As mentioned in Section 18.2.3, the tasks that users have to perform with the product are also an important consideration in that the sequence of use determines the product features that will be used. For example, the process of making toast does not use the crumb removal tray feature of the toaster. This feature might be used when occasionally cleaning the toaster, and the frequency of this task would be much lower than making toast. Consider the fragment of a task description for making toast in Table 18.3. It is evident that the greater level of detail in the task description exposes fundamental user actions required to perform the higher level tasks of making toast. We now consider the specific sensory, physical and cognitive demands made on users (Figure 18.5).

Table 18.3. Fragment of task analysis for making toast

2. Set toast heating level ...	2.0 *Understand* next action is to set toasting heat level 2.1 *Locate//Recognise* toast control 2.2 *Understand* what it does/how it works (level settings) 2.3 *Search* for required setting 2.4 *Choose* required setting 2.5 *Move hand to/Reach* to control 2.6 *Grasp* control (one handed operation) 2.7 *Rotate* control to required setting 2.8 *Release* control

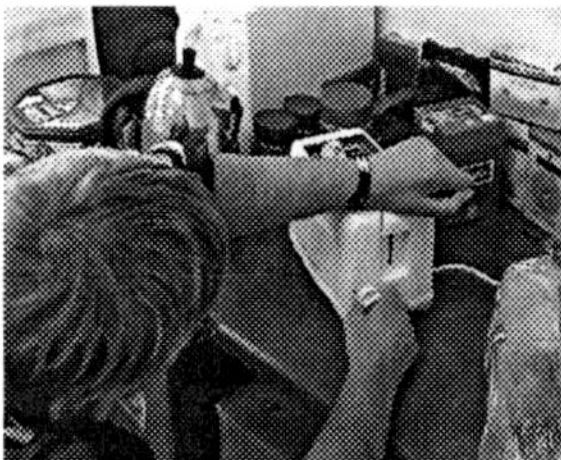
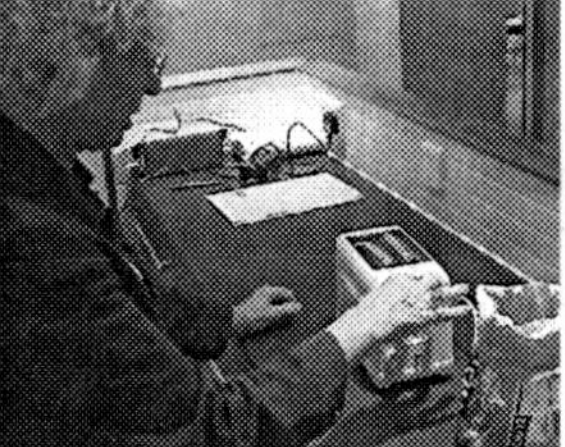
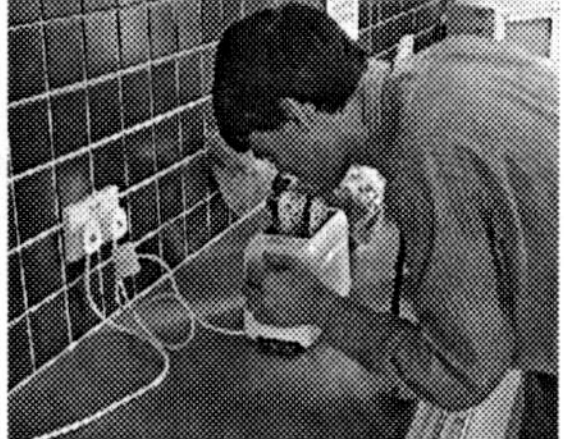

Figure 18.5. Video stills from toaster observational study for three users: a female wheelchair user, an older female user and a visually impaired male user

18.3.1 Sensory Demand

In terms of sensory demand, the male user with a visual impairment in Figure 18.5 had to move his head very close to the heating rotary control in order to see the numerical text labels. This is in part due to the placement of the control on the side of the product and also the size of the lettering on the rotary control. In general, users will move closer to the product or bring the product closer to their eyes if they cannot see text or symbols. These sensory displays on the product can be evaluated in terms of acuity, contrast sensitivity, visual field and colour vision required (assuming a general operating distance). By mapping sensory displays on the product to the estimated levels of acuity, contrast sensitivity, visual field and colour perception in the population, it is possible to estimate the level of exclusion that takes place. Furthermore we can also calculate scores for all the sensory displays on the product in terms of how much demand they place on users' visual capability.

18.3.2 Physical Demand

For physical interaction with the toaster, users are required to move their hands around the toaster (movement demands) or move the toaster itself, grasp and touch the toaster chassis and various controls (the slider handle, rotary heating control and the stop button). Users also need to exert the required forces in order to move the slider handle in a linear downward motion; the heating control in a rotary motion and the stop button with a linear finger depression. Finally, the physical dimensions of user and product must match in terms of finger, hand and arm lengths and sizes. The environment where the product is placed also plays a significant role in imposing reaching and movement demands. However, these are mostly beyond the control of the product designer and common environmental conditions can be assumed.

18.3.3 Cognitive Demand

Cognitive demands of products include requiring the correct mental model for operation. Similar to the conceptual model postulated by Norman (1999), this corresponds to beliefs about how the product works that arise out of design features and goal-based interaction. For this relatively simple toaster, the number of controls and available options is very small. Visually, the toaster appears very simple and allows for the functions of heating toast at a particular setting, and ejecting/stopping the toaster at any time. Users understood at first glance that the slider on the right of the toaster needs to be depressed to start the toaster and pressing the stop button stops and ejects the toast while bread is heating. Because there are only three controls that change the state of the toaster (the slider handle, rotary heating control and the stop button), there are no complex symbols, layouts or large number of controls to place knowledge, memory or search demands on users. Users also had the correct procedural mental model for operating the toaster, knowing that they must first set the heating level and then depress the handle to start the toaster toasting.

18.3.4 Coping Strategies and Affordances

In looking at the first and second video stills in Figure 18.5, the users used different fingers or parts of the hand to depress the slider handle – sometimes one finger, sometimes two fingers or the edges of the hand. Users with capability limitations typically employ coping strategies in order to operate different interfaces. Learning how various users cope with various interfaces can lead to design improvements. However, because coping strategies can be quite varied from person to person, we opt for a practical approach considering the most common forms of interaction.

Following Norman (1999), we can utilise affordances as another useful concept that can be applied to the analysis of product interfaces. An affordance is an attribute of a design feature offering, providing or furnishing the user with something. Hartson shows how this concept has informed usability and user-product interaction analysis such as AVANTI (Rizzo, 1997; Hartson, 2003) and includes sensory, physical and cognitive affordances as being properties of product interfaces that allow the user to perform sensory, cognitive and physical actions. A measure of how well the interface affords these actions to a particular user determines the usability of the interface. Thus the grippability, slidability and pushability of the slider handle are relevant physical affordances at "able-bodied" capability levels but are also applicable to more impaired interactions.

18.4 Conclusions and Further Work

This paper highlighted some weaknesses of empirical evaluation approaches and previous capability scales used in inclusive design evaluation. We proposed the system requirements for calculating improved scales of capability-demand interaction. To implement such a system it is necessary to develop a usable, systematic description of product interfaces. A simple toaster was used to illustrate various dimensions of product demand and how these product attributes combine to form a demand profile of the product. The comparison of the product interface demand profiles against capability scales is proposed as the overall framework for developing an inclusive evaluation method.

Once the evaluation scales are fully developed and tested, the scales and supporting data can be implemented as a software evaluation tool that can aid the evaluation process. Algorithms for calculating accessibility scores and comparing different products will also be implemented and tested iteratively in parallel with the scale development process. Appropriate visualisation techniques are also under development which will aid designers in visualising product accessibility dimensions using various multidimensional graphical techniques.

18.5 References

Clarkson PJ, Keates S (2003) User capabilities and product demands. In: Proceedings of INCLUDE 2003, Royal College of Art, London, UK

Dong H, Keates S, Clarkson PJ (2002) Inclusive design diagnosis based on the ONS scales? In: Proceedings of CWUAAT'02, Cambridge, UK

Hartson HR, Andre TS, Williges RC (2001) Criteria for evaluating usability evaluation methods. International Journal of Human-Computer Interaction 13(4): 373–410

Hartson HR (2003) Cognitive, physical, sensory, and functional affordances in interaction design. Behaviour and Information Technology 22(5): 315–338

Keates S, Clarkson PJ (2002) Defining design exclusion. In: Keates S *et al.* (eds.) Universal access and assistive technology. Springer, London, UK

Keates S, Clarkson PJ (2003) Countering design exclusion: an introduction to inclusive design. Springer, London, UK

Keates S, Clarkson PJ (2004) Assessing the accessibility of digital television set-top boxes. In: Keates S *et al.* (eds.) Designing a more inclusive world. Springer, London, UK

Kondraske GV (1995) A working model for human system-task interfaces. In: Bronzino JD (ed.) The biomedical engineering handbook. CRC Press, Boca Raton, USA

Langdon PM, Keates S, Clarkson PJ (2004) New cognitive capability scales for inclusive product design. In: Keates S *et al.* (eds.) Designing a more inclusive world. Springer, London, UK

Martin J, Elliot D (1992) Creating an overall measure of severity of disability for the office of population censuses and surveys disability survey. Journal of the Royal Statistical Society, A, 155(Part 1): 121–140

Martin J, Meltzer H, Elliot D (1988) OPCS surveys of disability in Great Britain. Report 1 – the prevalence of disability among adults, HMSO, London

Norman DA (1990) The design of everyday things. Doubleday, New York, USA

Norman DA (1999) Affordances, conventions and design. Interactions 6(3): 38–42

Persad U, Langdon PM, Clarkson PJ (2005) Assessing user capabilities from small scale samples. In: Proceedings of HCI International 2005, Las Vegas, USA

Rizzo A, Marchigiani E, Andreadis A (1997) The AVANTI project: prototyping and evaluation with a cognitive walkthrough based on the Norman's model of action. In: Proceedings of DIS'97, Amsterdam, The Netherlands

Smith S, Norris B, Peebles L (2000) Older adult: the handbook of measurements and capabilities of the older adult data for design safety. Department of Trade and Industry, London, UK

Semmence J, Gault S, Hussain M, Hall P, Stanborough J *et al.* (1998) Family resources survey, Great Britain 1996-97. DSS, Corporate Document Services, UK

Stanton N (1998) Human factors in consumer products. Taylor and Francis, London, UK

Chapter 19

Investigating the Role of Experience in the Use of Consumer Products

T. Lewis, P.M. Langdon and P.J. Clarkson

19.1 Introduction

Many products today are laden with a host of features which for the majority of users remain unused. Worse still, they bewilder and confuse the user into struggling to use the simple features for which the product was devised (Norman, 1988). This is especially true for elderly users where the prominence of cognitive impairment is higher and the cognitive demand; particularly on memory, is high. Products typically created by male, youthful, designers focus more on packing features within the product frame and functionality than on ease of use (Keates and Clarkson, 2003).

Effective usage of appropriate labelling and symbology is relevant to making a product easier to use (Nielsen, 1993). Beyond this, once the user has learnt how to use the product, suitable cues must exist such that the time required to re-learn the product on a subsequent usage is far shorter (Norman, 1988).

A range of products was tested across a spectrum of users. Products chosen vary from portable devices such as digital cameras to motor vehicles. Users were given a set of tasks that aimed to represent common everyday tasks as well as more uncommon functions. The users were chosen to cover a representative sample of society and included users with a range of impairments. This paper outlines the preliminary results from trials with a motor car.

19.1.1 Inclusive Design Aims

Inclusively designed products tackle the disparity that has arisen from a design culture dominated by young, non-disabled, males. Most products fit the stereotype of their designers, ignoring an increasing number of users who vary from mild to severe impairment and corresponding disability in society. Products meeting the ideals of inclusive design aim to minimise the number of person excluded (Keates and Clarkson, 2003).

19.1.2 Motivation from Previous Usability Studies with Symbols

A study by the primary author into the feasibility of customisation in videocassette recorders (VCRs) amongst elderly users exposed an unexpected result. Over 80% of the participants failed to recognise the common triangle and square symbols representing the play and stop functions. This was surprising as the symbols are unanimously used, not only within the VCR market but also extensively across DVD, CD and cassette players and all devices used for the playback of media. Whilst the elderly users' knowledge of such devices would be more limited than that of younger users, they had clearly been exposed to the symbols in the past (Lewis and Clarkson, 2005).

Whilst the bulk of inclusive design research has so far made significant progress in providing advice to designers on overcoming problems relating to physical and sensory disabilities, there is limited progress relating to cognitive impairments and learning issues. "Simulation kits" can, to some extent, provide the designer with an experience of having a wide range of physical and sensory disabilities, but the nature of cognitive problems and previous experience makes it significantly more complicated to give the designer an accurate empathy (Cardoso *et al.*, 2004).

19.2 Background

Guidelines relating to usability and human factors research exist in different forms from several different academic centres across the world. The TRACE Center (1992) published its guidelines relating to many different product types in the 1990's. The detailed section relating to consumer products contains vast amount of information aiming to cover displays, auditory signals, button forms and more. For those designers specialising in Assistive Technology, this is ideal. EDC research into promoting inclusive design has found that designers who create products for the mass-market need short, sharp advice (Dong, 2004).

USERfit was born from a European Commission initiative to promote 'design for all'. Its nine-stage methodology aims to introduce assistive technology awareness throughout the design process. Whilst already established at providing the designer with a framework to consider impaired users, it still offers more scope for guidelines that can assist the designer in specific impairments (Poulson *et al.*, 1996).

Analysis from user trials can often describe many of the problems with a particular product by considering the errors the user makes. Various classifications exist which attempt to break down the type of errors that can be made. Ryu and Monk's (2004) model explores the relationship between the user's "goal", "action" and "effect" and the errors that can occur between these in the cycle of interaction. Norman's (1988) "slips" also covers a scheme of errors of interest that break down similarly to those occurring between "thoughts" and "actions". Both schemes are relevant to the analysis of product learning but require augmenting with an additional experience focus to produce a classification that is not overly restrictive. Cognitive walkthrough approaches emphasise the goal structure of a user engaged in exploratory learning (Polson *et al.*, 1992) that is more sympathetic with the assessment of product interfaces that we are trying to achieve and may provide a framework for categorisation of interaction problems.

19.2.1 Product Design Advantages

Several commercially available products to have adopted the inclusive design ideals include BT's Big Button phone, the Ford Focus and OXO Good Grips kitchen utensils. Their success can be attributed to using inclusive design to consider both able and disabled users in their specification, developing a product that is usable by those with impairment without adding stigmas that would discourage able users. Furthermore, the increase in usability makes them more attractive to those fully able users.

The Big Button Phone primarily tackles sensory problems of reduced vision and hearing and the Good Grips utensils aim to solve manual dexterity issues. Products that lighten the cognitive load required to operate them offer even greater opportunities to include users with cognitive disabilities but also attract those without (Keates and Clarkson, 2003).

19.2.2 Cognition of Memory and Learning

Research in Human Factors Engineering uses complex models that subsume well-understood functions and processes in cognition while summarising decades of experimental evidence. For example, a model based on the human information processing approach to cognition and constructivist theories of visual processing would include memory functions such as Sensory memory; Short term memory (STM), Working Memory (WM); Long Term Memory (LTM), as well as memory models implying processes, such as Categorical Memory, and Prospective Memory, (Figure 19.1). It would also assume a central executive and executive functions, as well as binding processes to co-ordinate these (Baddeley, 2000). It would include parallel and serial selective attention; response selection; sensory cognition and visual search, reasoning, comprehension, language understanding and visual-spatial reasoning. Such a model (*e.g.* Wickens and Holland, 2000), assumes a complex relationship between attentional resources and cognitive processing, such that search, retrieval from memory and response selection are generally characterised as a sequential activity whose properties are approximated by a limited capacity processing system with parallel capability.

The difficulty with such models lies in the complex nature of the relationship between attentional resources and memory (*e.g.* Meenowa *et al.*, 2004). The cognitive system may operate slowly in an information-rich environment or may be equally at home in a time-limited, response or control environment. Familiarity with the experimental background of modern Cognitive Science is a prerequisite for easy interpretation of the performance of individuals in complex tasks, and this has been most effectively employed in human factors investigations of complex control activities such as piloting an aircraft (*e.g.* Kroft and Wickens, 2002). To provide guidance for the design of products for daily domestic use may not require such a complex understanding and could be managed by directing attention to well-understood, fundamental functions in cognition.

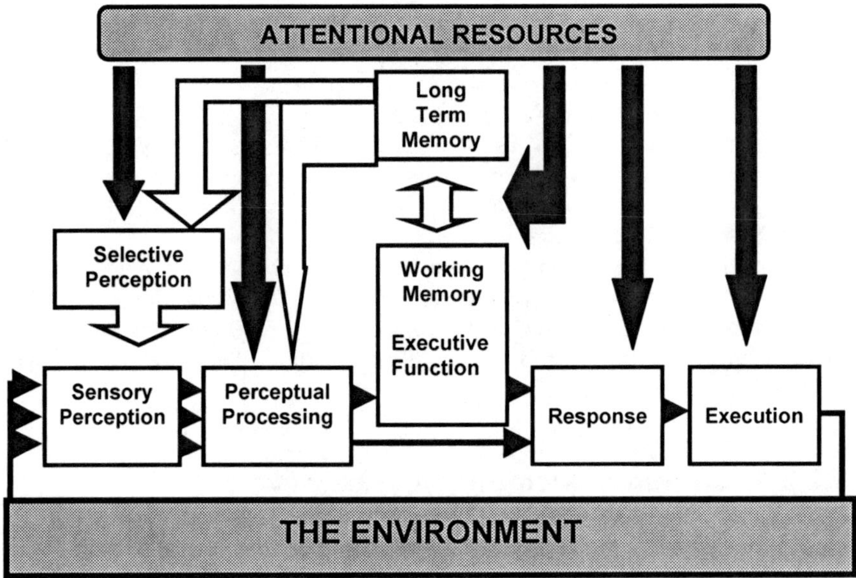

Figure 19.1. Simple cognition model

This simple cognition model approach provides an understanding of how the mind responds to a stimulus. Sensory organs perceive stimuli from the real world; many are ignored, flowing straight through the central executive causing little, if any, attention and no action.

If the central executive decides to act upon a stimulus, then it must refer to its memory. Long-term memory stores episodic and autobiographical experiences from the past. The central executive can check whether a stimulus has been experienced before, what the resulting actions were and whether the effects these had on the real world were the intended ones. The form of the stimuli will vary according to the situation; for a product this might be a symbol, in a conversation it would be a correspondent's words and other situations may include auditory alarms, temperature change, and touch and feel. The similarity of the stimuli to what has been experienced before will affect the speed and efficiency of the retrieval from the long-term memory for a given attentional context.

Working memory is for storing items whilst the central executive considers them. Processing in the central executive and use of the working memory have limits to both the amount of information they can handle and the speed of working. Attempts to exceed either of these will normally result in an incorrect conclusion, inappropriate action and ultimately slips, lapses and errors (Reason, 1990; Polson *et al.*, 1992; Meenowa *et al.*, 2004).

19.2.3 Experience

Experience is also a critical factor on how easy a product is to learn. All products make some reference to either previous generations or products from different families. Products that use this to help users make a reference to the same function on another device with which they are familiar should out-perform those that make no such association or worse still, make a different or incorrect reference (Sudjianto and Otto, 2001).

Memories relating to the experience of products will be stored in the long-term memory, and the ability of the central executive to find the relevant knowledge will depend on the cues provided and the amount of previous experience. The more times a user has completed an interface task the faster this process will become as the user progresses from novice to expert.

19.2.4 Pilot Studies

A procedure to run experiments on a number of products was developed through a number of pilot studies. A mobile phone was first trialled on a range of users completing a set of tasks, including everyday functions such as writing a text message and adding a contact to the phone book, through to more complex options such as changing the time. Users were asked to vocalise their thinking as they completed the task (concurrent protocol). It was later decided this would probably cause interference in their completion of the trial so a retrospective protocol was used. Users' experience of mobile phones was extensive and there was a large variation in the layout and menu arrangement of all the features and functions throughout the market.

The **iRiver** mp3 player was a compromise between an unfamiliar interface and familiar symbolic and semantic references in the labelling. The model chosen had high functionality but was also very compact. This led to a small number of buttons but a high modality, causing a significant cognitive load in the learning process. The modality problems led to the users having difficulty that was characterised by frequent errors and searches for feedback from the interface.

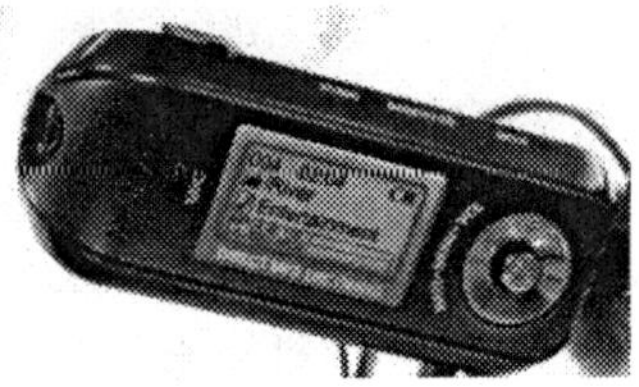

Figure 19.2. iRiver mp3 player

The pilot trials developed an awareness of the style of trial, the time a user would be happy to invest, the type of product and the procedure for capturing and analysing the data. The information learnt was used to select products that could be analysed and of which users would have a sufficient lack of experience for further trial.

19.3 Method: A Motor Car

The task list aimed to include functions that covered a spectrum from everyday functions to barely-used operations. Controls that caused the car to move were excluded, so the task list had to consider procedures involving the lighting, wipers, heating, seat position, and so on. The users tested varied in both age and sex but an additional difference unique to this product was also explored. The users were either drivers or non-drivers, the drivers having gone through a learning process after the age of 17. It was expected that although the non-drivers would have little, if any, driving experience, there would be some experience effects through watching drivers whilst being a passenger.

Users were given the task list, below, and asked to read it through before attempting the trial, allowing questioning relating to comprehension problems with the tasks but not on how to complete the tasks. On completion the user was then shown the recording and asked to provide a protocol, explaining their interpretation of their mental process. This was recorded separately. Follow-up questions were asked after the user's commentary. Task list – Car Trial:

1. Settle into car and adjust seat position to reach pedals comfortably
2. Switch front windscreen wipers on and then off
3. Activate rear windscreen screen-wash
4. Switch headlights on
5. Switch full beam on
6. Switch all lights off
7. Turn heated rear windscreen on and then off
8. Open front passenger window and then close

Fifteen users were sampled in the first phase, of whom eight were males and seven females. The age range varied from 20 to 60 with clustering at the limits. The data was analysed focusing on the errors, time taken to complete tasks and the users' interpretation of their problems. Organised in a spreadsheet, this allowed easy comparison between users and provided the means to spot trends across age, sex or driver/non-driver factors. Protocols were segmented and split into the following broad categories:

- No response – fear of damage, lack of knowledge
- Previous memory (proactive interference)
- Difficulty with feedback
- Comprehension failure
- Memory failure
- Repeated Trial and Error

19.4 Results and Analysis

The car provided interesting results since the users not only varied between drivers and non-drivers but also two users who were learning to drive and a motorcyclist who did not have a UK car license. A sample analysis is included in Figure 19.3 below showing how the trial was broken down into each event, the cognitive area involved, the product's response/feedback and whether this represented an error by the user:

						Manipulation	
Time	difference	action	sub-action	Product response	Cognition	Intentional	Random
0	6	adjust car seat	moves seat rise lever	seat slightly rises higher	•		•
6	6		moves seat forward lever	seat moves on rails	•	•	
12	4		check pedals		•		
16	3	front wipers	examines wiper stalk		•		
19	6		turns on front wipers	wipers move		•	
25	5		turns off front wipers	wipers stop		•	
30	4	rear screen wash	turns on front wipers	wipers move			•
34	8		activates front screen wash	screenwash fires			•
42	6		turns off front wipers	wipers stop		•	
48	2		passes on rear screen wash		•		
50	4	headlights	examines lights stalk		•		
54	2		turns sidelights on	sidelights and icon light		•	
56	1		turns headlights on	headlights and icon light		•	
57	4		turns lights off	lights and icons off		•	
61	9	beam	turns sidelights on	sidelights and icon light			•
70	3		turns sidelights off	lights and icons off		•	
73	1	lights off	passes on beam		•		
74	7	heated rear windscreen	examines lights stalk		•		

Figure 19.3. Analysis of a typical trial by a user, aged 20, female, non-driver

19.4.1 Observations

Many users found the multifunction stalks on which the lighting and wiper controls were mounted confusing. Most checked both before touching either, indicating that the labels on each were inconclusive. Notwithstanding, many rechecked each side when having to perform the alternate task possibly showing that the first task didn't provide them sufficient feedback to be convinced they had it correct.

Several users had problems with feedback on elements including lighting and heating controls. This was partly because the trials were completed during daylight and under timed conditions. In the case of the former, the user was unable to tell if the headlights were on without leaving the vehicle and for the latter, there was insufficient time to judge if the heating changes had taken effect. In both cases there were icons that lit up to indicate that the function was switched on but this was not sufficient to enable the users to complete the task.

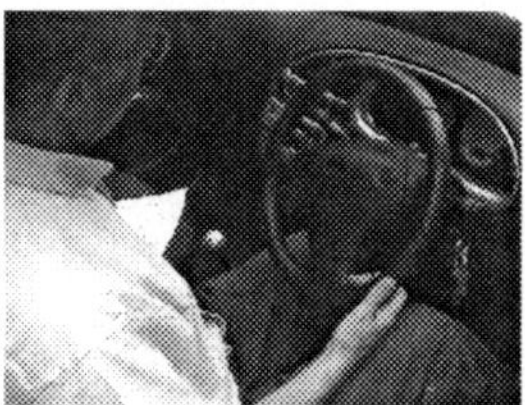
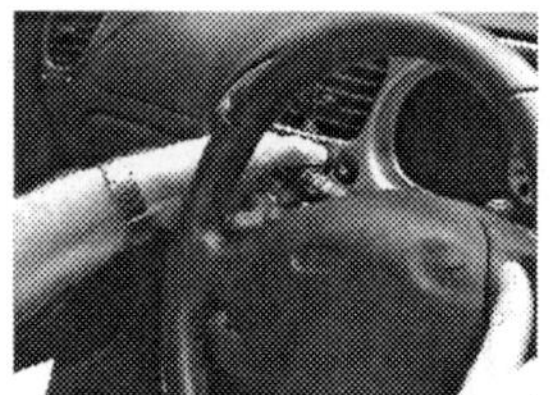
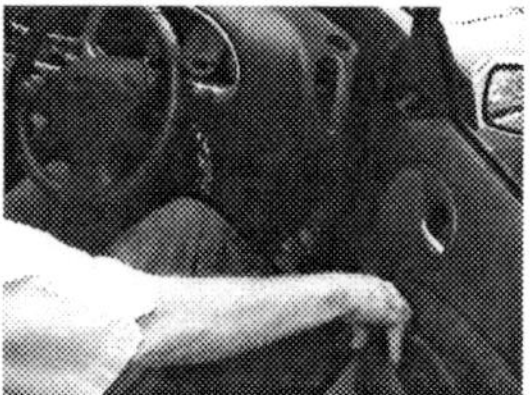

Figure 19.4. A male driving user during the trial (aged 55)

Window controls were generally well understood: no users experienced problems opening the passenger window from the driver's seat. This demonstrates the effect of experience in that both drivers and non-drivers will have performed this function before.

There was a clear distinction in results between those who could drive and those with no experience. Non-drivers passed on many more tasks and their errors tended to focus on repeated trial/error and "no-response" due to lack of confidence to use the trial and error strategies. Drivers generally passed all the tasks but those who owned European cars took longer than those with American models probably because the car used was American.

19.4.2 User Commentaries

A selection of the users' quotes from their commentaries is included below;

"...and then I tried to work out how to get the rear ones [wipers] I thought that you had to turn the thing [stalk] but you just had to move it, and I worked it out in the end."

female, 20, non-driver

"...I thought it was going to break it off, the thing [stalk], because I knew you had to turn it but it felt if you turned it, it would break off. So I just left it."

female, 20, non-driver

"the windscreen wipers - I wasn't sure which side to go because, I think, its different in my car" "The heated rear windscreen - I know the symbol so that was easy to find, although it was in a different position to my own [car]."

female, 54, driver

"Rear windscreen wash was obvious to me because it's very similar to my car."

male, 55, driver

19.4.3 Discussion

Observations and the commentaries both indicated a problem with the stalk controls. Whilst these are clearly highly developed arrangements by manufacturers and are unlikely to change in the short term, there are more general standards that could be used for design. Designers should avoid using similar controls but with a different arrangement of functions within the same product family.

Feedback is vital to the ability of a user to learn a device. Where it is lacking, learning will take longer. For the drivers, this lack tended not to cause errors, but did cause significant time delays; for the non-drivers, the problems led to errors. For the multifunction stalks, the error would be classified as due to proactive interference and the feedback would simply be labelled as a lack of feedback in a simple cognitive approach. Norman's (1988) classification scheme focuses mainly on faults from the user rather than failures within the product and hence has insufficient focus on product features to distinguish the effects of controls. Alternatively, Ryu and Monk's (2004) cyclic interaction theory would have them both described as "goal-action" errors either from weak affordances of the correct action – for example, the symbols present on stalks are inadequate indicators of function – or strong affordances of an incorrect action – for example, similarities in the shape and action of the buttons for the heated rear windscreen and the fog lights. Each approach provides a different element of the sort of description needed for aiding the process of devising guidance for product design.

19.5 Conclusions

There are some clear indications from the car trial on the effects of layout of controls, lack of feedback and lack of confidence that the product won't break if a trial and error strategy is adopted. The preliminary results are beginning to show consistency in the effects of experience, as might be expected. Further trials will be carried out with further populations of users and on other products across the consumer product spectrum, to develop and extend the results and the guidelines produced from specific cases to the more general. Guidance will be developed on how knowledge of the target users' experiences can be used to design a product that will be both quick and easy to learn.

19.6 References

Baddeley AD (2000) The episodic buffer: a new component of working memory? Trends in Cognitive Sciences 4: 417–423

Cardoso C, Keates S, Clarkson PJ (2004) Comparing product assessment methods for inclusive design. In: Keates S *et al.* (eds.) Designing a more inclusive world. Springer, London, UK

Dong H, Keates S, Clarkson PJ (2004) Industry perceptions to inclusive design. In: Proceedings of Design Engineering Technical Conference, Utah, USA

Keates S, Clarkson PJ (2003) Countering design exclusion: an introduction to inclusive design. Springer, London, UK

Kroft P, Wickens CD (2002) Displaying multi-domain graphical database information: an evaluation of scanning, clutter, display size, and user activity. Information Design Journal 11(1): 44–52

Lewis T, Clarkson PJ (2005) A user study into customising for inclusive design. In: Proceedings of INCLUDE 2005, Royal College of Art, London, UK

Meenowa J, Langdon PM, Furner S (2004) Using haptic displays for workload reduction and inclusive control. In: Proceedings of HCI International 2004, Las Vegas, USA

Nielsen J (1993) Usability engineering. Academic Press, London, UK

Norman D (1988) The design of everyday things. Doubleday, New York, USA

Polson PG, Lewis C, Rieman J, Wharton C (1992) Cognitive walkthroughs – a method for theory-based evaluation of user interfaces. International Journal of Man-machine Studies 36(5): 741–773

Poulson D, Ashby M, Richardson SJ (eds.) (1996) USERfit. A practical handbook on user centred design for assistive technology. HUSAT Research Institute for the European Commission

Reason R (1990) Human error. Cambridge University Press, UK

Ryu H, Monk A (2004) Analysing interaction problems with cyclic interaction theory: low-level interaction walkthrough. PsychNology Journal 2(3): 304–330

Sudjianto A, Otto K (2001) Modularization to support multiple brand platforms. In: Proceedings of Design Engineering Technical Conference, Pittsburgh, USA

TRACE Center (1992) Accessible design of consumer products. Available at: http://trace.wisc.edu

Wickens CD, Hollands JG (2000) Engineering psychology and human performance, 3rd edn. Prentice-Hall, New Jersey, USA

Chapter 20

Software Co-design with Older People

G. Dewsbury, I. Sommerville, P. Bagnall, M. Rounceﬁeld and V. Onditi

20.1 Introduction

> *Our Lives are getting evermore technologically demanding. The number of skills necessary to participate fully in modern-day society are continually increasing and so is the expected level of technological know-how.*
>
> (Keates and Clarkson, 2003)

In a world that is orientated towards the healthy and the younger person, designers have been reticent to design inclusively. This is beginning to change due to the overwhelming evidence that older people are likely to be a considerably larger proportion of the population by the year 2020. The notion of 'inclusive design' emphasises the importance of social, human factors in system use. Designers should recognise that solutions devised on the basis of inappropriate investigative strategies and techniques can be debilitating and dis-empowering (Lebbon *et al.*, 2003). Consequently, when considering technology design for older people, traditional technological approaches need to be complemented by detailed investigations into everyday life and user needs, involving the users themselves in the process of investigation and requirements specification as a feature of co-development or 'co-realisation' (Hartswood *et al.*, 2002). Current practice still considers older or disabled people as specific groups set apart from the norm of society for which special demands are placed on the designer in order to produce one-off designs. This paper reports on the development of a person-centred approach to developing a communications and virtual games platform for older people to use in their own homes. We initially consider the methods and research process used in determining people's needs and aspirations, and consider our adoption of cultural probes as a facilitator in this exposition. The paper reflects on the implications of the design in relation to inclusivity and demonstrates that the approach adopted by the research team considered the participants from a person-centred perspective.

Our research originated as part of the DIRC (http://www.dirc.org.uk/) initiative, a multi-institutional investigation funded by the EPSRC on dependability in computing systems. On this project, we worked with a number of older people in the community to design a technology system that would be suitable for them. In the process of this investigation, our original conception of designing some form of smart or ubiquitous home was found to be misguided by the participants whose concerns were mundane, relating to undertaking everyday household tasks and avoiding isolation and loneliness. Our investigations found that, even in housing specifically designed for elders with available social facilities, older people still felt lonely and isolated. We observed how they used the television as a means of avoiding their isolated experience, the television taking the place of the lost partner, in a silent static form.

As a response to the isolation that many of the participants were experiencing, we started to investigate how we could make use of computer-mediated communications as a way to facilitate non-intrusive, informal communications between older people. Critical to this was the development of a system that was both usable by people suffering from many of the normal infirmities of old age and which did not look like a conventional computer with all of the preconceptions that this entailed. We therefore decided to base the support system on tablet computers – simple A4-sized devices which are light and portable and which do not require keyboard skills for interaction. This system is still in development, and crucially the participants have been used to inform the design process throughout.

20.2 Eliciting User Requirements

One of the most complex and time-consuming elements of designing for people is actually the requirements process. In order for the final design to be accessible to and actually used by the target group, it is critical that this group or person is fully engaged with the design process. The process of designing for individuals is a strong tradition at Lancaster University's computing department where a number of technology designs have been undertaken using small groups or individuals. Our methods tend to use a very small group to define the problems in a general sense and to give grounding to the process. The design is roughed out and then presented to a wider group for comments. This leads to the next design stage which is more concrete, and through successive iterations the design becomes more refined and detailed. At several points through the process the emerging design is presented back to the larger group. This process means that needs and aesthetic qualities can be embedded in the design.

Sensitivity to the feelings of the participants who agreed to be part of our studies required a range of sympathetic data gathering techniques. The starting point for this data gathering was the use of cultural probes (Gaver *et al.*, 1999, 2004) which we adapted for our purposes to provide us with design data (Crabtree *et al.*, 2003). Some participants agreed to keep personal diaries of their daily activities. All were also supplied with Polaroid cameras and voice activated Dictaphones in a Cultural Probe pack. In addition to these items, the packs consisted of a disposable camera, photo album, visitors book, scrapbook, post-it notes, pens, pencils and crayons, a set of postcards addressed to the researcher and a questionnaire. We are currently using a probes pack containing, rather than the other cameras, a digital camera, which only requires a 'point and click' to take a picture.

A key feature of our probes was their mundane nature, as they consisted of every-day artefacts which were easily obtained from any main street and therefore were all familiar to the participants. Even if they had not used the devices previously, they had at least been aware of them and considered them to be ordinary (Cheverst *et al.*, 2003). The lack of the 'wow factor' actually assisted in the uptake of the probes. The participants felt happy to engage with the everyday artefacts whereas it is uncertain how they would have responded to-out-of-the-ordinary articles.

The probes have been trialled by Lancaster in a number of settings and projects, including with adults with cognitive impairments in a halfway house, which resulted in the development of a SMS interactive display board that is used by the staff and the residents, as well as pill dispensers (Kember *et al.*, 2002; Cheverst *et al.*, 2003; Clarke *et al.*, 2003; Fitton *et al.*, 2004). The probes have also been adopted for disabled and older people living in the community to assist in designing assistive technology solutions as well as within a sheltered home for older people in which an evaluation of their current technology was undertaken (Dewsbury *et al.*, 2004). For each occasion, the probes were developed and adapted for the people who would use them. For the older people the Dictaphone and cameras were chosen, as they are easy to use as well as requiring little dexterity by the participants. The questionnaires were specifically written for each group to reflect their living styles and their possible lifestyles.

Probes were handed out in ones and twos as special packages, attempting to make the person who has the probes package feel special and important. The probes were left with the participants for a period of time that they determined but no less than two weeks in order for the research team to get a clear idea about their routines and patterns of behaviours. In all groups, the probes were greeted with interest as well as a degree of concern. For many of the older people the probes seemed to be something they would do, but only as they were involved in the research project, although over time the concerns of many of these people were diffused by the participants who had completed the probes and found them both fun and enjoyable.

Our own approach to the use of cultural probes embodies much of Gaver's (Gaver *et al.*, 1999) original propositions but we deviate in a number of significant practices. Entry into the participants' home is often difficult to negotiate. The probes act as a mediation tool between the participants and the research team as well as actively involving and engaging them from the off. This facilitates the sometimes difficult negotiations involved in accessing participants and 'bringing them onboard' so to speak. The probes are used not as artistic works designed to promote inspiration in the minds of participants and researchers but rather as grounded artefacts that enable the participants to share personal aspects of their lives with the researchers. Therefore the probes act as a negotiation and navigation tool to direct the researchers through the layers of personal and sensitive topics that the participants wish to share with the team. Our emphasis is not placed on older people answering specific questions by using the probes. This is undertaken through the qualitative questionnaire, and rather we provide the probes with as little instruction as possible in order for the participants to generate the data on their own terms.

The probes were well received: in the community, the six older people from a north east town were given and returned the packs, and in the sheltered home where the researchers were present for a longer period, fifteen probes were given and returned. Not all the elements of the probes were fully completed, and the amount of completion seemed to be proportionate to the participant's impairments. The greater their impairments, the less probe material returned completed. This is not wholly surprising, but allowed us to redesign the probe contents each time. Certain items were never used by participants in certain groups including the Dictaphone (A Sony M-430), which might be because this was given to older people who did not like to hear their own voices and therefore felt embarrassed. Also even though the Dictaphone was small and required little skill to use, the buttons were small and not clearly illustrative of their use, requiring considerable strength to push them all the way down to start the recording process. It is not always easy to be sure why certain items were not taken up whilst others were used effectively. The results from the probes have been discussed elsewhere (Cheverst *et al.*, 2003; Clarke *et al.*, 2003; Crabtree *et al.*, 2003)

Although our expectations of the results from the probes were limited we had not anticipated that loneliness and isolation were felt as acutely as they turned out to be. Even in residences where the participant lived with a group of other people of similar ages there was a significant amount of loneliness present. If their friends had family or relations for the weekend, it meant the person might spend the weekend without seeing anyone else even though people were next door to them. The main requirement therefore was a tool to facilitate and support communication. Informal communication was essential as participants did not want to feel obligated to make a formal connection with the other person (Bagnall *et al.*, 2004). The question that struck the design team was how to enhance informal communication by enabling older people to engage with a piece of technology and use it as a communication tool.

20.3 Promoting Communication

Whilst designing a computer based communications tool, one of the first questions that have to be answered is what hardware platform is appropriate for older people? There are several competing considerations. Many older people are technophobic, unfamiliar with computers or somewhat reticent about learning to use them, so the system should be as natural and simple to use as possible. Some older people have limited space in their homes, especially those living in sheltered accommodation, and they might find difficulty in reading small typeface and thus require a larger screen.

The available hardware options are currently desktop PCs, Laptops, Tablet PCs, and handheld devices such as the Palm. Desktop PCs are importable and take up too much space, Laptops can be awkward to use, and some older people might find them too heavy to move around comfortably. Palm sized devices can be too small for some older people to read easily. This leaves Tablet computers as the best options, specifically slate style tablet PCs. The one actually being used weighs 1kg, which we have found to be generally acceptable. Tablet PCs have few hard buttons, which have been disabled so that they do not produce confusion with the users. Input is via a stylus, which is somewhat familiar to older people since it looks and behaves in a similar way to a simple pen (Figure 20.3). Tablets also generally include 802.11 wireless networking, which makes connecting to the Internet physically much easier than having to deal with wires.

For the software platform, the most obvious choice might be to build applications on a standard OS such as Windows XP. However, these contain very large numbers of interaction options, which can make them hard to learn and could be overwhelming for some users. Instead it was decided to build a system which sits on top of Windows XP, but provides a simpler user experience, hiding the complex Windows GUI.

The software design that emerged over a period of a few months was inspired partly by instant messenger systems. The ability to see quickly who else was available on the system was seen as an essential to allow discrete communication. An important aspect of instant messenger is the ability to advertise "status". Typically systems allow "Online", "Busy" and a small number of other status messages. However, it seemed unnecessary to restrict older people to such a small set of status messages. Instead a simpler and richer option was to provide a small area where they could write a message which would be seen by all their friends and family. Messages can be changed just by wiping the area clean by tapping a button and writing the new message. Early trials of this feature suggested this was both simple enough to be readily understood, and enjoyed. This design meant that most of the screen would be taken up with an "address book", but since the device is focussed on communication, and helping people to see who else is available to communicate with, this has proven a successful option.

The other feature present on the first screen (known as the CHOOSER) is a list of activities (Figure 20.1). Currently we have only tested only one, namely CHAT, which allows synchronous written communications (Figure 20.2). To start an activity the user taps on the activity button and on the other participants, and then taps "Start". The start button allows users to change their minds if they accidentally tap the wrong thing, and also makes the order in which choices are made (people first or activity first) more flexible.

The chat activity design is aimed at being simple but powerful. It presents an interface which looks much like a shared whiteboard. The various participants can write and draw, and see each other's writing and drawing almost instantly. This design helped to avoid a problem with instant messenger style applications, namely threading. In instant messenger it is common (Isaacs *et al.*, 2002) to see more than one conversational thread. For younger people who are familiar with the technology this is generally acceptable, but even for them is can become confusing and hard to follow. The shared whiteboard style design avoids this since responses are likely to be made near to the original utterance, so the spatial layout can be used to alleviate the confusion threading might cause.

Once the whiteboard fills up the design relies on a paging system. This was instead of a scrolling system, which can be physically awkward with a stylus. Making sure the software was designed in a way that was appropriate for the hardware was a major consideration of the design.

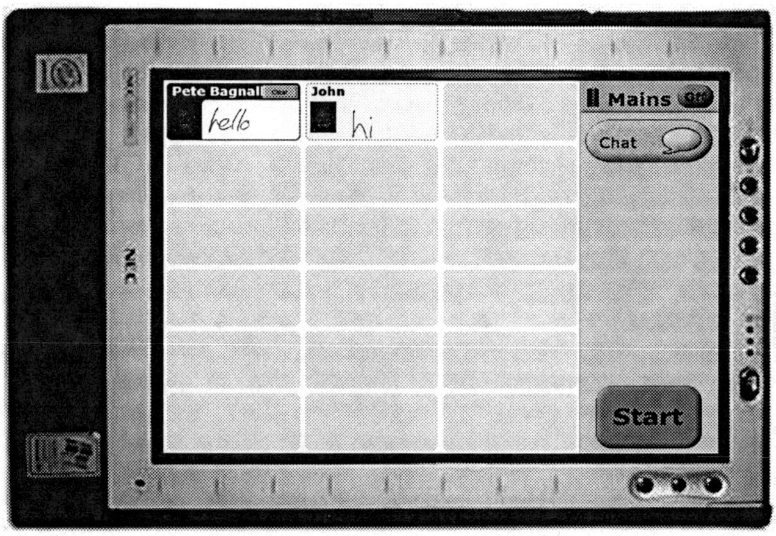

Figure 20.1. The CHOOSER

Through discussions with the participants we were informed that entering data via keyboard and a mouse was not suitable for many people: we therefore opted for a stylus entry. The tablet comes with two styli. One fits into the casing of the tablet, but unfortunately is too thin for the majority of our participants. The larger stylus however, being about the same dimensions as a biro, was found to be acceptable by the participants. The stylus has a button which has been disabled as this caused an unnecessary complication for some users and therefore acts just like a normal pen. This was found to be a useful analogy for the participants to use in order to get over certain technophobic issues.

To operate the system, all the user is required to do is turn it on and then the choices are simple choices. To illustrate, Figure 20.1 shows the CHOOSER page displaying the other network users, the computer recognises this automatically, and then the user is required to choose what application they wish to use, in this case they have a choice of one: 'CHAT'. By selecting who they wish to chat with, selecting CHAT, and then pressing the start button they go into chat mode. They are then prompted to write an optional invitation. Once they have written this the invitation is presented to the people they selected who can then accept or reject the request and if accepted the CHAT mode begins (Figure 20.2). The simplicity of the platform is its strength: it allows the users to do many things but the options are always the minimum possible for the task. As we add more applications the

CHOOSER page will fill up on the right hand side but the choices will always be limited and there are a maximum number of add-ons that are allowed. Therefore, if users wish to undertake a series of complex tasks such as email, accessing the web, editing and managing photographs *etc.*, they have the option of choosing from a limited number of tasks.

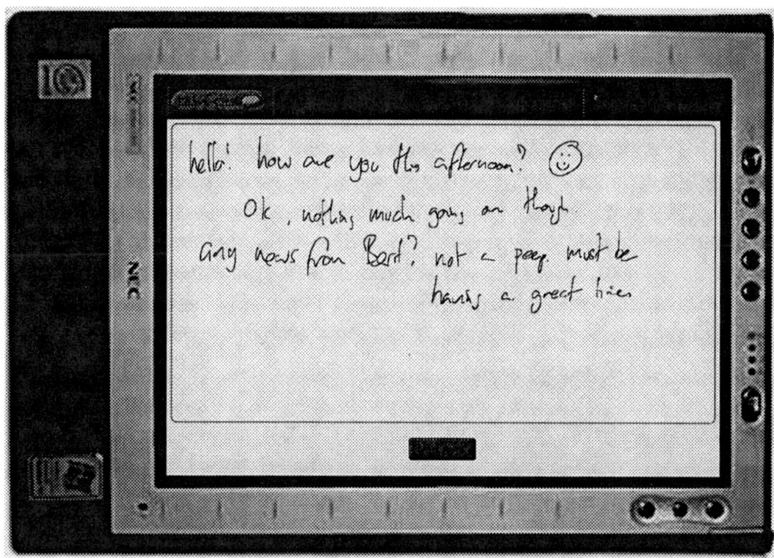

Figure 20.2. The tablet in "CHAT mode"

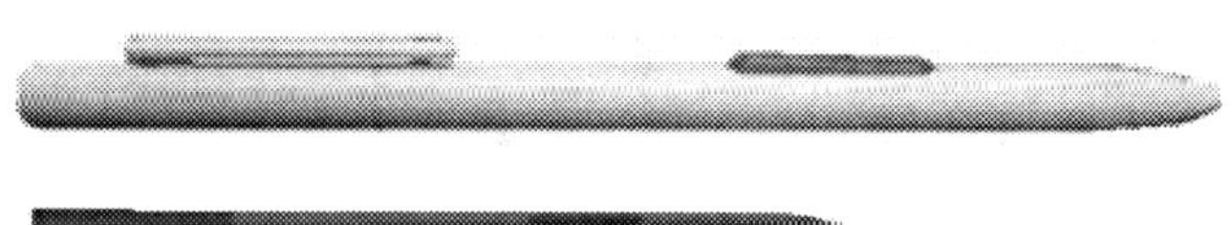

Figurer 20.3. The different styluses proved a useful comparisson

20.4 Communicating through Games

Surprisingly or at least surprising to anyone who spends any time observing the daily life of older people, little attention has been paid to the role of games in the lives of older adults. Our ethnographic studies have highlighted how games – crosswords, card games, Scrabble *etc.* – were an important and valued part of their individual and social lives. Games appear important for a number of reasons. Firstly, as a source of entertainment and enjoyment; secondly as a mechanism to develop new social contacts and reinforce existing friendships; and finally as therapy, slowing down memory loss and maintaining motor skills as well as improving self-esteem and independence. We see particular benefits arising where games facilitate social interaction. To support both individual and social game playing requires research to help understand the most effective means of interaction with computing platforms and how we can support, for example, people talking during games, player awareness, coordination, *etc*.

The ability to chat between older people allows for informal communication. Clearly the application allows users to write and draw pictures, thereby giving alternative communication methods, but the chat application is simply designed to facilitate interaction which could then continue in other ways (phone, visits, *etc*.). We are now investigating how to supplement this system with applications that allow closer engagement with the computing platform and have begun to develop a card games platform for the tablets which will enable a range of multi-player games to be played with each player interacting with other remote players through their tablet computers. Note that this is not, primarily, a system to play games with a computer – rather, it is a means for people who may be housebound to play games and interact with their friends. As Lindley (2004) suggests:

> *"games are not simply games, they are perhaps more accurately referred to as ludic systems, systems that integrate game play with other formal systems of interaction and time structure."*

We have therefore designed the games support facilities to be flexible and to allow games to be played as determined by the tablet users (Figure 20.4).

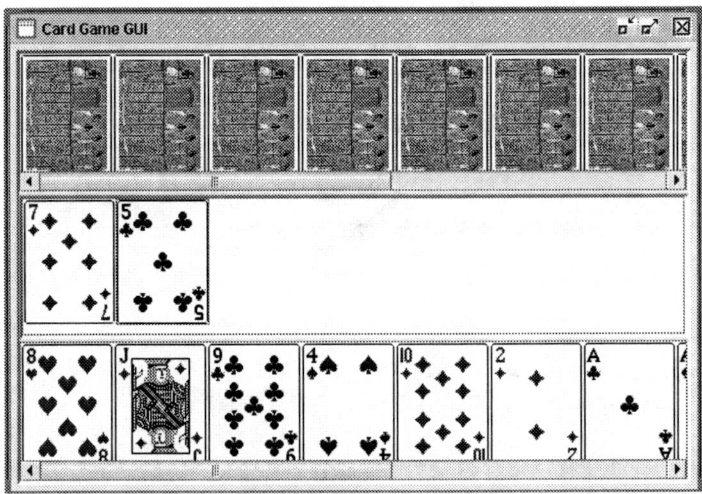

Figure 20.4. The FREECARD games console with all hands showing

Existing computer based games remove decisions on rules from human agents to computer systems. While this approach has its own merits, it denies the player the flexibility of traditional games. Ideally, it would be nice to provide unintelligent game objects which allow players to manipulate the objects during the play. For example, it should be possible to play a different game with the same game objects as with their physical counterparts. Our approach strives to achieve the flexibilty exhibited by traditional games through decoupling rules from game objects and transferring them to the player. The consequence of the rule transfer is the need to support communication between players. Clearly doing this by written contact is not feasible as it would be too cumbersome; we are therefore using Skype (http://www.skype.com/) to allow real time verbal communications between the tablet users. The tablets already have basic microphones and speakers built into them and therefore this voice transfer application achieves a basic connection between users relatively simply. This allows social chat between players as well as discussions on the game itself. Games therefore perform a number of interesting communicatory functions, in that they provide a source of entertainment and an event; this is a social event, which can also be a learning event and a physical event.

20.5 Concluding Thoughts

The development of the tablet platform and applications continues, the tablets successfully transmit the writing from one to another in real time and the chat and games applications have been developed to a beta stage. They are currently being tested with participants in their own homes. The technology developed is a direct result of the co-working relationship that the team have built up with the participants. Without them there would be no design, and without them there would be no improvements. Throughout the course of this research we have attempted to work with the participants as equals in the project and reflect their wishes in the final designs. It has been a learning experience for all members of the team. We also see that although the applications have been developed on tablets for tablet PCs there is no reason why we cannot use them on standard computers. Similarly, although the applications were developed for older people by older people, there is no reason why they cannot have as much worth with other people in the wider world.

20.6 Acknowledgements

This work has been partially funded by Microsoft Research as part of their ‘Create, Play and Learn’ collaborative research programme and partially funded by the Engineering and Physical Sciences Research Council as part of the DIRC Interdisciplinary Research Collaboration. We would also like to thank Age Concern Carnforth, MHA Care Group, Age Concern Barrow in Furness and Dundee Social Work Department for their assistance in this study.

20.7 References

Bagnall P, Dewsbury G, Sommerville I (2004) Easy for everyone: using components to offer specialised interfaces for software. In: Proceedings of the 1st HEAT: The Home and Electronic Assistive Technology Workshop, Computing Department, Lancaster University, UK

Cheverst K, Clarke K, Dewsbury G, Hemmings T, Hughes J *et al.* (2003) Design with care: technology, disability and the home. In: Harper R (ed.) Inside the smart home. Springer, London, UK

Clarke K, Cheverst K, Dewsbury G, Fitton D, Hemmings T *et al.* (2003) Cultural probes: eliciting requirements for dependable ubiquitous computing in the home. In: Proceedings of HCI International 2003, Crete, Greece

Crabtree A, Hemmings T, Rodden T, Cheverst K, Clarke K *et al.* (2003) Designing with care: adapting cultural probes to inform design in sensitive settings. In: Proceedings of OzCHI 2003, University of Queensland, Brisbane, Australia

Dewsbury G, Clarke K, Rouncefield M, Sommerville I (2004) Depending on digital design: extending inclusivity. Housing Studies 19(5): 811–825

Fitton D, Chevherst K, Rouncefield M, Dix A, Crabtree A (2004) Probing technology with technology probes. In: Proceedings of the Equator Workshop on Record and Replay Technologies, Equator IRC, London, UK

Gaver WH, Dunne A, Pacenti E (1999) Design: cultural probes. Interactions 6(1): 21–29

Gaver WH, Boucher A, Pennington S, Walker B (2004) Cultural probes and the value of uncertainty. Interactions XI.5: 53–56

Hartswood M, Procter R, Slack R, Voß A, Buscher M *et al.* (2002) Co-realisation: towards a principled synthesis of ethnomethodology and participatory design. Scandinavian Journal of Information Systems 14(2): 9–30

Isaacs E, Walendowski A, Whittaker S, Schiano DJ, Candace K (2002) The character, functions, and styles of instant messaging in the workplace. In: Proceedings of CSCW 2002, New Orleans, Lousiana, USA

Keates S, Clarkson PJ (2003) Countering design exclusion: an introduction to inclusive design. Springer, London, UK

Kember S, Cheverst K, Clarke K, Dewsbury G, Hemmings T *et al.* (2002) Keep taking the medication: assistive technologies for medication regimes in care settings. In: Keates S *et al.* (eds.) Universal access and assistive technology. Springer, London, UK

Lebbon C, Rouncefield M, Viller S (2003) Observation for innovation. In: Clarkson PJ *et al.* (eds.) Inclusive design: design for the whole population. Helen Hamlyn Research Centre, Royal College of Art, UK

Lindley C (2004) Ludic engagement and immersion as a generic paradigm for human-computer interaction design. In: Proceedings of the 3rd International Conference on Entertainment Computing, Technical University Eindhoven, The Netherlands

Chapter 21

Creating User Centred Creative Design Tools for the Packaging Industry Using Video Ethnographic Research Techniques

K.J. Gough

21.1 Introduction

This paper describes a two-year research project to develop creative design tools for designers and marketers to explore user needs and aspirations for packaged products. The work was carried out at the Helen Hamlyn Research Centre in collaboration with the Faraday Packaging Partnership between October 2003 and October 2005. During the research, three case studies engagements were completed with Marks & Spencer, Coors Brewers and Nestle. During each case study, observational research was conducted with key consumers from each brand owner or retailer. The project developed user-centred, video ethnographic research techniques to enable in-house groups to conduct research with key consumers. Importantly, the video material captured provided consumer insight into the use of packaging in the context of the store and the home. Results from the research informed the development of design tools tailored to each company. These tools were aimed for use by designers, marketers and innovation managers, to enable them to evaluate how a pack performs to meet consumer needs and aspirations.

21.2 Research Question

Packaging design, manufacture and supply has evolved greatly in the last twenty years. Using ethnographic research techniques to investigate user interactions with packaging is a valid step in acquiring knowledge about the needs and desires of consumers. The consumers' relationship with the pack starts long before they open it. From the moment it is seen on the supermarket shelf, to the point when it is used in the home, packaging gives off visual clues. Previous research with older users and packaging, at the Helen Hamlyn Research Centre, identified that if consumers encountered a new pack format of which they had no previous experience, they would not engage with it. This could happen in the supermarket or at home. The first year research, a pathfinder study, investigated “How can the visual communication of food packaging enhance the consumer’s ability to access its contents?” Marks and Spencer provided access across their food categories to enable research with key consumers. (See Tannahill, 1988; Crow, 2003).

21.3 First Year User Research Strategy

Each household featured independent, active consumers with access to supermarket food over several shopping trips during the week. Each user was given £25 of Marks & Spencer vouchers to spend during their observed shopping trip. They were asked to purchase at least a few components for a meal they would normally consume, and were free to purchase other items. After the trip, they were observed at home, unpacking and storing their purchases, and then cooking a meal. With the user’s consent, each engagement was recorded using a video camera. Analysis and editing of the ethnographic video footage taken during each engagement, aimed to identify issues on two levels. Firstly, identifying the visual clues contained in existing packaging that worked well to inform use. Secondly, identifying potential areas of need, around which design briefs for new packaging could be generated. Observations and interviews captured each user’s relationship with a product in the context of store and home. By shadowing consumers as they shopped in store, unpacked and prepared food at home, insights emerged around key interaction points with packaged products, providing evidence of aspects of visual communication throughout the lifecycle of a pack (Figure 21.1). (See Miller, 1998; Jordan, 2000).

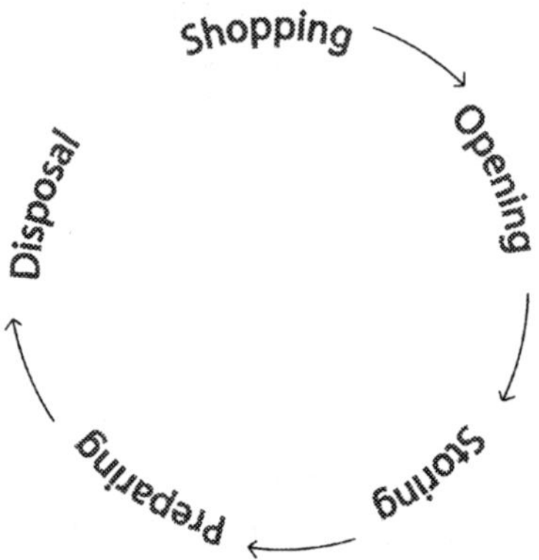

Figure 21.1. Lifecycle of a pack

21.4 Design Tool

A design tool was developed as a direct result of the research. The tool formalises key insights from the research and provided an intuitive visual interface for evaluation and comparison (Figure 21.2). It is aimed to aid designers and marketers to make design decisions about how packaging should communicate visually, physically and cognitively. Each segment of the tool represents a consumer consideration or decision during the lifecycle of a pack. The questions posed by the tool relate to five different packaging roles: shop and select; open and access; store and decant; prepare and consume; and dispose and recycle. A scoring system for the questions enables a spidergram to be generated for each assessed pack. Analysis of the shape provides a measure of inclusivity – the fatter the shape, the more the visual communication of the pack is working right through its lifecycle to aid ease of use. Video material from research forms insights to prompt the creative design process. (See Tufte,1983; Newark, 2002).

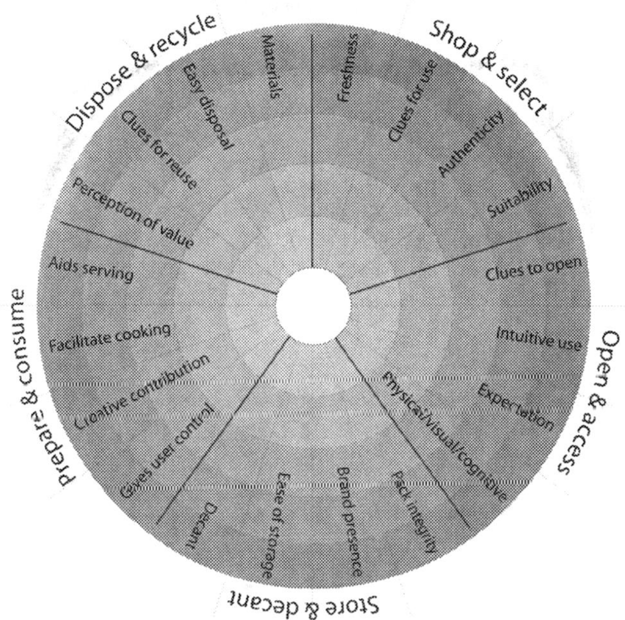

Figure 21.2. Design tool

21.5 Packaging Design Exemplars

The collated insights from the video research were translated to design briefs that formed the basis for packaging design exemplars to illustrate and support the user-centred design tool. Two example designs, based on adaptations of existing Marks & Spencer food packs for salad and courgettes, were generated as concept computer renderings to support the design tool (Figure 21.3). Before and after designs were scored using the design tool to show how application of simple design changes can improve the usability of a pack (Figure 21.4). (See Cawthray and Dennison, 1999; Calver, 2004).

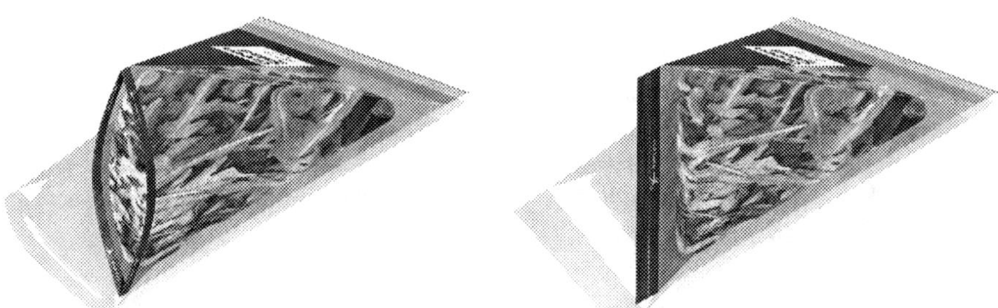

Figure 21.3. Computer rendering of packaging examples, developed to illustrate the design tool process

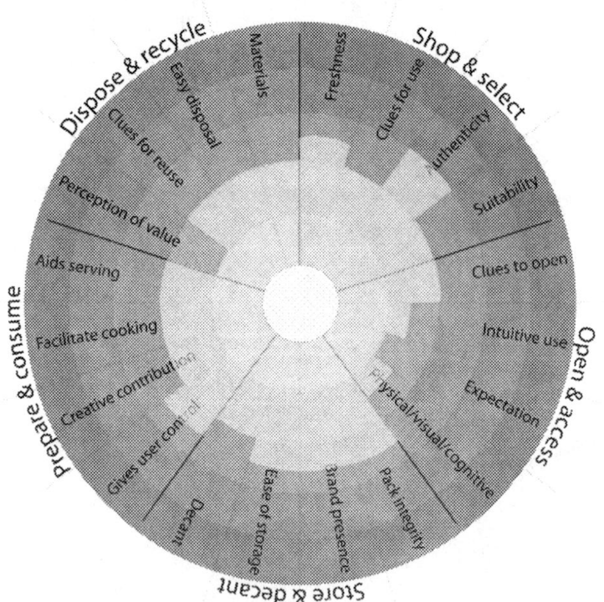

Figures 21.4. Example of vegetable packaging evaluation using the design tool

21.6 Developing the Methodology

The second year of research built on the first year pathfinder study, to develop the research and design methodologies used in the design tool. Importantly, the work engaged with two further brand owners to explore how the design tool could be adapted to their needs and transfer knowledge. The two industry case study engagements, conducted with Coors Brewers, Burton-on-Trent, and Nestlé Packaging Technology Centre, York, provided application for the design tool on live industry packaging design projects. The research conducted with users focused on individual brand product lines. Importantly, the work sought to refine the process of developing a design and research tool, tailored to a company's individual needs and core brand values. The research also sought to explore ways in which the consumer could be represented in the design and marketing process.

21.6.1 Second Year User Research Strategy

An important development in year two was adapting research methodologies to augment and complement existing market research techniques that could inform the design tool. Coors and Nestlé chose specific products in their brand range. During the pathfinder study, user engagements had a pure research remit, and were free to range across all food categories following the key users involved. During the second year, order to focus on specific brand products, it was necessary to develop more formalised user research engagement, which included:

- accompanied shopping trip in a supermarket used regularly
- observations of unpacking and storing purchases
- interview in the home
- cupboard tour

Users were again identified based on each brand's customer segmentation groups. Both companies attended research with users. All aspects of the engagement with consumers were captured on video. (See Laurel, 2003).

21.7 Outcomes

During the second year the user research enabled the design tool to be developed, refined and tailored to represent each brand's consumer needs and aspirations. The design tool was also evaluated for:

- benchmarking existing packaging or competitor packaging
- fostering user research techniques within a company
- evaluating packaging design concepts and prototypes
- providing iterative packaging design process in conjunction with user research.

At a meta-level, the second year of research developed a methodology for working with brand owners and retailers in order to develop and tailor individual consumer-centred design tools. The project identified a time and cost-efficient process for research methods that engage users in order to generate insights, which feed directly into the creative design process. The project sought to understand how the gap between consumer-led research and company understanding and perception of consumers could be bridged.

21.8 References

Calver G (2004) What is packaging design? Rotovision

Laurel B (ed.) (2003) Design research methods and perspectives. MIT press, Cambridge, USA

Cawthray R, Dennison E (1999) Packaging prototypes. Rockport Publishers, USA

Crow D (2003) Visible signs. AVA publishing, Switzerland

Jordan P (2000) Designing pleasurable products. Taylor and Francis, London, UK

Miller D (1998) Material culture. Why some things matter? UCL Press, Taylor and Francis, London, UK

Newark Q (2002) What is graphic design? Rotovision SA

Tannahill R (1988) Food in history. Penguin, London, UK

Tufte ER (1983) The visual display of quantitative information. Graphics Press, Cheshire, USA

Chapter 22

Differing Perspectives on Telecare: An Attitudinal Survey of Older People, Professional Care Workers and Informal Carers

J. Hanson and J. Percival

22.1 Introduction

This paper reports findings from a recent attitudinal survey into the implementation of telecare. Providing older people with increased independence to better meet their needs forms a key part of the care policy agenda in the UK. In this respect, telecare is perceived to be an important new weapon in the armoury of support services, which should result in fewer older people requiring institutional care and more remaining independent in their own homes for longer than would otherwise be the case. This paper evaluates such objectives by reporting on attitudes towards telecare among the contributors to 22 focus groups, comprising 92 older people, 55 professional stakeholders and 39 carers, that were convened in three different regions of the country as a precursor to telecare service development. The results suggest that the respondents' attitudes and views were shaped by prior knowledge of conventional service delivery in their local area, and that future expectations and requirements in respect of telecare will be informed by wider perceptions about the extent to which community care should operate as a preventative strategy or as a mechanism for crisis management.

22.2 Context for the Study

This presentation concerns findings from a six month long study of older people's attitudes to telecare, carried out between June and December 2004. The study provides input to a much larger, ongoing research consortium that commenced in October 2003 and is due to report in late 2006. The overall aim of the consortium is to understand the opportunities for and barriers to 'mainstreaming' telecare services in the homes of older people. A major impetus for the formation of the consortium was the inclusion of three project partners where telecare installations are planned to take place in people's homes within the life of the project. All of the consortium's work, including the results of the attitudinal survey that is presented here, is therefore taking place in Barnsley, South Buckinghamshire and Plymouth, where these field sites are located. These are very different regions of the country, so the attitudinal survey reported below has taken evidence from older people living in a very wide variety of circumstances.

Promoting the independence of older people forms a key part of the UK government's health and social care agenda, and new care delivery models supported by information and communication technologies (ICTs) are being developed to assist in realising this goal, (Audit Commission, 2004, Barlow *et al.*, 2005b). Telecare is one such model that uses ICTs to bring health and social care directly to the end user, by providing safety and security monitoring, physiological health and activity monitoring, and information to people in their own homes (Barlow *et al.*, 2005a).

A typical telecare service involves a system that connects sensors of various kinds that are dispersed in the homes of (or worn by) an older person, to a call centre. The sensors are either activated by the user, or raise a passive alert, by recognising and responding to a change in the user's status, such as a fall, in real time. The alert goes to a call centre, which then triggers a response that may involve informal carers, resident or mobile support staff or an emergency service, as required. Other sensors monitor people's patterns of activity over longer periods to detect changes in behaviour that could indicate a decline in health, known as lifestyle monitoring. In some ways, current versions of telecare are simply an extension of the existing community alarm services, (Brownsell, 2000). The difference is in the growing use of ICTs to deliver more control over the domestic environment and provide reassurance for those being cared for and their carers, as well as allowing carers to receive advance warning of trends to intervene in a more timely fashion.

Like many initiatives in the field of e-health, the promotion of telecare is a product of an ageing society. Whilst the numbers of older people are increasing, concerns have been raised that the numbers of informal carers are declining. For those informal carers who remain, carer stress is an important and a major reason older people are admitted to a residential care home. The UK government wishes to plug this emerging 'care gap' by providing telecare services to all those who need them by 2010 and to that end it has recently invested £80 million to stimulate the uptake of telecare services (Department of Health, 2005). The stated objective is to support more older people in their own home for longer, by preventing unnecessary hospital admissions, permitting earlier discharges, and reducing the numbers admitted to residential care (Aldred *et al.*, 2005). Less often stated, though no less pressing, is the need to reverse the escalating costs of healthcare.

22.3 Mainstreaming Telecare in the Homes of Older People

Evidence is now accumulating which demonstrates the efficacy of telecare in reducing hospital admissions and unblocking beds (Louis *et al.*, 2003; Bayer *et al.*, 2004). But, whilst there is widespread experience of telecare through pilot and demonstration projects, its introduction into mainstream care practice has so far proved far more problematic. The mainstreaming of telecare is falling well short of the government's aspirations, and there is now doubt as to whether their targets for 2010 and beyond can realistically be achieved.

Recognised barriers to take-up include: overcoming the organisational complexity of the care delivery process; aligning differences between organisational cultures and values; demonstrating the efficacy of telecare through systematic cost/benefit analysis; and building the business models that link the different actors in the supply chain into a transparent pricing mechanism (Barlow *et al.*, 2005b). However, an important reason for telecare's failure to make it into the mainstream is not technological failure, but its unacceptability to users (Sixsmith and Sixsmith, 2000; Levy *et al.*, 2003, Demiris *et al.*, 2004).

UCL was therefore tasked by the consortium to benchmark the opinions and attitudes to telecare of a broad cross-section of older people living in the three regions, before the planned interventions took place. We also wanted to compare older people's views with those of local health and care professionals involved in service delivery to older people in their own homes, and informal carers who were looking after older people. Later on in the project, we shall compare these 'ambient attitudes' with those of individuals who are personally involved in the field sites, immediately before installation and after nine months living with the technology.

22.4 Research Methodology

At the time when this study was undertaken, telecare was a new service and there were no existing telecare installations in any of the three fieldwork areas, so we could not assume any prior knowledge of the service. It was therefore necessary to explain the concept in a standard way, using simple terms that connected with people's previous experiences. To this end, we developed three 'scenarios' that described people living in realistic situations where telecare could provide a solution to a perceived need, such as forgetting to turn off the bath taps, waking and wandering during the night, recurrent problems with falling in the home or neglecting to eat regular meals, to a more general disengagement from society resulting in social isolation.

We developed the scenarios in such a way that they could be discussed in small focus groups of about six to eight people. Separate groups were formed of older people, professionals and carers, so that each could speak freely. After the discussion, we asked for a show of hands in response to nine questions, intended to gauge people's opinions about different aspects of telecare. The answers could then be compared by group and by region, to see whether opinions concurred or differed according to people's roles or circumstances. Before starting fieldwork, ethical approval for the study was gained from UCL's Committee on the Ethics on Non-NHS Human Research.

Our target was to recruit thirty older people, fifteen carers and ten professionals from each area. In the end, twenty-two focus groups were convened, five with carers, seven with professionals and ten with older people, leading to a final sample size of one hundred and eighty-six individuals, see Table 22.1 below. The youngest older people were in their late fifties, and the oldest participants were aged over one hundred. Service providers were drawn from the sectors of health, social services and housing, as well as local older people's charities and voluntary organisations. The numbers of respondents to the question and answer sessions (nQ) do not equate with the totals taking part in focus groups, as, due to other commitments, a few participants had to leave the focus groups after the case study discussions and before the question and answer event took place. The percentage figures have been calculated just on the basis of those people who actually gave answers to the questions.

Table 22.1. Participants in the attitudinal survey, by region and by type of respondent

	Older People	**Carers**	**Professionals**	**Total**
Barnsley	36	11	11	58
S. Bucks	25	27	13	65
Plymouth	31	17	15	63
Total	92 (nQ=91)	55 (nQ=53)	39 (nQ=37)	186 (nQ=181)

Focus group discussion was recorded and subsequently analysed for content. In addition, the answers to the standard questions were analysed by type of respondent and by region. The answers to each of the nine questions could be 'yes', 'no' or 'do not know'. From these, simple percentages were derived, which made comparison easier than the raw data that contained widely different numbers of individuals and so could be more easily compared to establish if clear numerical differences emerged between the groups or across regions.

22.5 Findings

The answers to each of the nine questions are set out below, see Table 22.2 and 22.3. Whilst some questions elicited a strong degree of agreement among sub-groups and between the respondents from Barnsley and those living in Plymouth and S. Bucks, areas of strong disagreement also emerged (The figures from these two regions were broadly similar and so, for brevity, they have been amalgamated.). This is all the more surprising, because the initial impression we had when carrying out fieldwork was that the focus group discussions were rather predictable and picked up on a few, well rehearsed themes, suggestive of rather uniform findings across all twenty-two focus groups involved. These included the use of technology, autonomy, privacy and the potential loss of human support, as well as issues of choice and self-determination, assessment, back-up services and cost.

In response to the first question, "Do you feel you understand the purpose of telecare and how it works?", 100% of professionals, 99% of carers and 95% older people said 'yes', which is a good result as if they had not, it would have reflected badly on our presentation.

However, in answer to the second question, "Would you be happy to have such a service in your own home?", a clear difference emerged between professionals, carers and older people. 92% of professionals and 80% of carers said 'yes', whereas only 67% of older people agreed, showing that people who look after others are keener to see this service put into place than those who are receiving care. Interestingly, though, older people in Barnsley were more ready to accept the service than those from Plymouth and S. Bucks (81% as against 53%).

Question three, "Would you be confident to have your blood pressure etc. monitored electronically, as opposed to going to the doctor or having a community nurse visit you at home?", established that 73% of older people would, with respondents from Barnsley more ready to do so than those from Plymouth and S. Bucks, and 57% of carers agreed, which is interesting because the intention of the service is that they are one of the groups who ought to be reassured by this happening automatically. However, carers in Plymouth and S. Bucks were far less enthusiastic than any of the other groups involved (40%). Overall, 83% of professionals said 'yes', perhaps a lower percentage than their enthusiasm for the service in principle would have predicted, and moreover whereas 100% of the Barnsley professionals would be happy to receive this service, only 65% of professionals from Plymouth and S. Bucks agreed that they would have more confidence in telecare than a home visit.

The next question asked, "Do you think people with telecare will be able to stay in their own home for longer that those who do not?". 98% of older people thought so, as did 87% of carers, but just 41% of the professionals agreed, which is noteworthy as this is one of the main justifications for the technology. Here, however, the professionals who are responsible for commissioning the service are probably more conscious of the actual 'trigger factors' that prompt a move up the care ladder. There were no particularly marked regional differences in respect of this question, other than a slightly greater scepticism on the part of informal carers in Plymouth and S. Bucks as to the ability of telecare to prolong independence.

One explicit concern among older people is that telecare will be used by care providers as a substitute for home visits, and in response to a direct question "Will it reduce the need for face to face visits?", a profound split emerged among the older service users. Just 4% of older respondents from Plymouth and S. Bucks and 4% of their informal carers agreed with this proposition, whereas 94% of the older

Barnsley residents and 100% of their informal carers agreed with the proposition. Half of the professionals agreed, but the rest predicted that the need for face to face visits would actually increase with telecare.

Table 22.2. Responses to questions in Plymouth and S. Bucks

	Plymouth and S. Bucks								
	Older people (nQ=55)			**Carers (nQ=42**			**Professionals (nQ= 26)**		
Q.	Y	N	A	Y	N	A	Y	N	A
1	100%	-	-	98%	-	2%	100%	-	-
2	53%	29%	18%	60%	36%	4%	88%	4%	8%
3	71%	22%	7%	40%	50%	10%	65%	27%	8%
4	96%	4%	-	74%	7%	19%	46%	4%	50%
5	4%	96%	-	4%	91%	4%	46%	27%	27%
6	74%	22%	4%	69%	17%	14%	96%	-	4%
7	7%	82%	11%	2%	91%	7%	-	100%	-
8	51%	22%	27%	62%	24%	14%	92%	8%	-
9a	6%	87%	7%	17%	83%	-	23%	77%	-
9b	64%	27%	9%	76%	7%	17%	58%	38%	4%
9c	15%	80%	5%	17%	66%	17%	81%	15%	4%
9d	60%	25%	15%	21%	60%	19%	27%	73%	-
9e	71%	20%	9%	43%	38%	19%	92%	8%	-
9f	92%	4%	4%	31%	48%	21%	96%	-	4%
9g	87%	7%	6%	52%	-	48%	80%	12%	8%

Table 22.3. Responses to questions in Barnsley

	Barnsley								
	Older People (nQ=36)			**Carers (nQ=11)**			**Professionals (nQ=11)**		
Q.	Y	N	A	Y	N	A	Y	N	A
1	89%	11%	-	100%	-	-	100%	-	-
2	81%	6%	13%	100%	-	-	100%	-	-
3	75%	22%	3%	73%	-	27%	100%	-	-
4	100%	-	-	100%	-	-	36%	-	64%
5	94%	-	6%	100%	-	-	55%	-	45%
6	100%	-	-	100%	-	-	100%	-	-
7	14%	86%	-	-	100%	-	-	-	100 %
8	50%	44%	6%	9%	9%	82%	64%	9%	27%
9a	-	100%	-	-	100%	-	27%	9%	64%
9b	94%	-	6%	91%	-	9%	-	36%	64%
9c	19%	78%	3%	-	-	100 %	9%	27%	64%
9d	25%	53%	22%	-	-	100 %	-	36%	64%
9e	11%	67%	22%	-	-	100 %	36%	-	64%
9f	97%	3%	0%	-	-	100 %	36%	-	64%
9g	39%	36%	25%	-	-	100 %	9%	27%	64%

Question six sought views on the extent to which people are likely to be safer at home with telecare. Again, older people from Plymouth and S. Bucks were more doubtful. 74% agreed, whereas 100% of Barnsley informants agreed with this proposition, as did 98% of professionals across both regions. Moreover, only two thirds of informal carers in Plymouth and S. Bucks perceived that there would be a benefit in this respect, whereas all the informal carers in Barnsley felt that their loved ones would indeed be safer with telecare.

In terms of risk management, answers to question seven, "Should someone older and known to be 'at risk' ever be prescribed a package of telecare, 'for their own good'?" revealed that just 10% of older people agreed with this proposition. No professionals were prepared to recommend this, but remarkably whereas all the Plymouth and S. Bucks representatives declared a definite 'no' on ethical grounds, all the Barnsley ones abstained. Informal carers were also opposed to the imposition of telecare on an older person who exhibited 'risky' behaviour.

A spectre that emerged in all focus groups was that of 'Big Brother', so it is no surprise that, in response to the question, "Do you have any concerns about the kind of information on lifestyle patterns that telecare is able to gather about how people are living at home?", half of the older people in both regions said 'yes', as did 62% of carers from the south of England. Barnsley carers felt less able to decide, as 82% abstained on the issue. More interestingly, 78% of professionals also agreed, again showing that professionals in both regions are, at this point in time, slightly uneasy about the potential of the service to redefine the boundaries of what personal information should be available when making decisions about individual cases. A far greater proportion of professionals in Plymouth and S. Bucks had reservations (92%) than in Barnsley (64%).

The final question concerned the point in the transition, from being fully independent to being in receipt of a package of care services, at which people should be offered telecare. No older people in Barnsley and few in Plymouth and S. Bucks thought that telecare should be routinely offered at 65 (response 9a). The contributors to all the older people's focus groups agreed that this would be too soon. Informal carers echoed this view, but 17% from Plymouth and S. Bucks thought it would be appropriate, whereas 100% from Barnsley thought it would not be. Professionals in both regions took a different view, and nearly a quarter from Plymouth and S. Bucks (23%) and just over a quarter from Barnsley (27%) felt that telecare should be routinely offered at 65.

Nearly all older people from Barnsley (94%) thought that they should be offered the service if they were ill as did 91% of carers (response 9b), but none of the professionals who were engaged in service delivery in Barnsley thought this would be appropriate. 6/10 older people from Plymouth and S. Bucks thought they should be offered it if they were ill, as did three quarters of carers, and about the same number of professionals agreed.

Low numbers of older people in both regions thought telecare should be routinely offered to people in sheltered settings (response 9c), which is interesting as this is perceived by service providers to be a key target group. Our older informants felt that sheltered housing gave an equivalent service so that telecare was not necessary. 9% of Barnsley professionals agreed, and in this respect their views were more similar to older people, but four fifths of the professionals from Plymouth and S. Bucks thought that telecare should be a service for people in sheltered settings, precisely because people in sheltered housing had already put a foot on the 'ladder of care'. Carers were more divided on the issue; 66% of southern carers disagreed with the proposition that telecare should be offered to people in sheltered settings and all the Barnsley carers abstained.

A different kind of logic applied in respect of community alarm users in Plymouth and S. Bucks (response 9g), where there was agreement between users (87%) and providers (80%) that telecare was a legitimate extension of the existing service, but not in Barnsley where a smaller percentage of older service users (39%) and a very low percentage of those responsible for delivering support services in the community (9%) felt that possession of a community alarm was a valid reason for also offering telecare. Carers from Plymouth and S. Bucks were evenly split on the issue, but all the Barnsley carers abstained.

Despite reservations in focus groups, a far higher percentage of older people from Plymouth and S. Bucks (60% and 71%) thought telecare should be offered to people who might be perceived as vulnerable (response 9d, when living alone and response 9e, if suffering from dementia) than did their Barnsley counterparts (25% and 11%, respectively). The professionals in both regions were broadly in agreement with their respective client groups so the professionals were also strongly polarised in favour (Plymouth and S. Bucks) or against (Barnsley). Professionals in both regions saw telecare as having more to offer to dementia sufferers than to people living alone. Southern carers were more willing to express an opinion on these issues, but those from Barnsley were unable to make up their minds.

Telecare was considered as an alternative option to residential care by nine out of ten older people (response 9f). On the whole, the professionals from Plymouth and S. Bucks also felt it was appropriate to offer it in these circumstances, but most of the Barnsley ones did not. As before, informal carers were undecided. In effect, most older people in Plymouth and S. Bucks thought telecare should be offered in any situation that might be construed as adding to risk, as people could always refuse it, but not if they were obviously managing independently, and on the whole the service providers took a similar view.

22.6 Discussion

Older respondents from Barnsley seemed to have adopted a slightly different attitude to telecare to their peers in Plymouth and S. Bucks. Their attitude could be interpreted more as ‘crisis management’, in that they perceived that it could be useful when ill or at risk of going into a care home, but otherwise most people’s realistic assessment was that the situations described would not be assessed by their local care provider as a sufficiently high priority. This seemed to reflect a correct assessment of local health and social services priorities, as most professionals did indeed judge that telecare was not an appropriate service for most of the situations we suggested, and none of the situations we described in Q9 attracted more than one third of the professional vote in Barnsley.

Older people from Plymouth and S Bucks, on the other hand, seemed to be thinking of the service as more of a ‘preventative’ strategy, and so argued that it would be beneficial to be offered the choice of telecare in any situation where it might have the potential to reduce risk, and on the whole their local support services professionals also took the same view.

This difference of opinion is unlikely to have resulted from different states of prior knowledge about telecare, as nobody we spoke to knew much about it in advance of the study. On the contrary, most attendees had come to a focus group to find out more. Nor could these differences in voting patterns be explained by different group dynamics, as the sessions were run to a standard format and our initial analysis of the transcripts has confirmed that the discussions took a fairly predictable trajectory, raising similar points, observations and dilemmas for professionals and service users across all three field sites.

The differences in voting patterns therefore seem to have been produced by people's prior experiences of conventional health and social care service delivery in the three areas, and the assumptions, attitudes and values that shaped and underpinned the quality and availability of existing community support services. What has been identified is not so much a north / south divide, as different attitudinal differences that have more to do with local circumstances and broad geographic factors. However, this is an important finding in terms of the government's ambitions for telecare, for these attitudes will undoubtedly prove to be another intervening variable that should be added to the 'barriers to mainstreaming', discussed earlier.

If these findings have any degree of general relevance, then commissioning bodies that are operating in 'crisis management' mode will look to telecare to support a relatively small proportion of the older population in their region, and the devices they commission will be selected to alleviate very specific situations, like monitoring serious chronic health conditions. Older people's expectations are also likely to be lower, and so they may not push for a wider application of the service. It may be viewed more as a medical intervention, and the ethos could well be to adopt a 'medical' definition of need.

Where a 'preventative' strategy has been adopted by health and social services, we can expect telecare to achieve widespread acceptance and distribution among older people living independently in the community, with more interest in aspects like lifestyle monitoring that aims to detect small changes in behaviour that could be indicative of deteriorating health or quality of life, well before a crisis ensues. Perceiving this, older people are likely to demand a more comprehensive array of devices, insofar as they perceive these to enhance their safety and security in the home. It is likely that telecare will be seen as a lifestyle intervention, so the ethos is likely to follow a 'social' definition of need.

Both the demand for and the supply of telecare services is therefore likely to be influenced by how different actors and agents perceive the whole purpose of health and social care, particularly the extent to which it should function as a rapid response to an individual crisis or as a preventative service for everyone. In this respect, the government's aim to mainstream telecare will be affected by different perceptions of 'need', which result from these different paradigms and pre-structures at least as much as by individual choices and requirements.

22.7 Acknowledgement

The research for this paper was funded within EPSRC's EQUAL programme (grant number GR/S29058/01) and was carried out by the authors in collaboration with Imperial College London, Dundee University, Barnsley Hospital NHS Foundation Trust, Anchor Trust, Thomas Pocklington Trust and Tunstall.

22.8 References

Aldred H, Barlow J, Brownsell S, Curry R, Hawley M (2005) Gerotechnology – meeting whose needs? In: Proceedings of the 5th International Conference of the International Society for Gerontology, Nagoya, Japan

Audit Commission (2004) Implementing telecare: strategic guidelines for policy makers, commissioners and providers. Audit Commission, Public Sector National Report, London, UK

Barlow J, Bayer S, Curry R (2003) The design of pilot telecare projects and their integration into mainstream service delivery. Journal of Telemedicine and Telecare 9(S1): 1–3

Barlow J, Bayer S, Curry R (2005a) Flexible homes, flexible care, inflexible organisations? The role of telecare in supporting independence. Housing Studies 20(3): 441–456

Barlow J, Bayer S, Castleton B, Curry R (2005b) Meeting government objectives for telecare in moving from local implementation to mainstream services. Journal of Telemedicine and Telecare 11(S1): 49–51

Bayer S, Barlow J, Curry R (2004) Assessing the impact of a care innovation: telecare. In: Proceedings of the 22nd International Conference of the System Dynamics Society, Oxford, UK

Brownsell G (2000) Using telecare: the experiences and expectations of older people. Generations Review 10: 11–12

Demiris G, Rantz M, Aud M, Marek K, Tyrer H *et al.* (2004) Older adults' attitudes towards and perceptions of 'smart home' technologies: a pilot study. Medical Informatics and the Internet in Medicine 29(2): 87– 94

DoH (2005) Building telecare in England. Department of Health, Older People and Disability Division, London, UK

Levy S, Jack N, Bradley D, Morison M, Swanston M (2003) Perspectives on telecare: the client view. Journal of Telemendicine and Telecare 9: 156–160

Louis A, Turner T, Gretton M, Baksh A, Cleland J (2003) A systematic review of telemonitoring for the management of heart failure. European Journal of Heart Failure 5(5): 583–590

Sixsmith A, Sixsmith J (2000) Smart care technologies: meeting whose needs? Journal of Telemedicine and Telecare 6(Supplement 1): 190–192

Chapter 23

Away from Home (Public) Toilet Design: Identifying User Wants, Needs and Aspirations

J. Bichard, J. Hanson and C. Greed

23.1 Introduction

This paper reports back on EPSRC sponsored VivaCity 2020 research 'The Inclusive Design of Away From Home (Public) Toilets in City Centres' (Hanson *et al.*, 2004), previously presented at CWUAAT 2004. Since the introduction of the Disability Discrimination Act (DDA) in October 2004 providers of 'away from home' toilets have had to ensure that 'reasonable adjustments' have been made to overcome the barriers to access many disabled people face (DRC, 2002). The DDA's remit has included just about every feature of the away from home toilet, from the cubicle to the soap dispenser. This research has sought to understand the attitudes, perceptions, functional constraints and cultural and social requirements of all the stakeholders in the process, and will report on 'personas' that have been developed to convey design specifications to built environment professionals. Further investigations on current toilet provision based on design guidance laid out in the British Standard BS8300 have been evaluated using a 'toilet audit tool' in Clerkenwell, London. This tool has enabled the research to pinpoint areas within the accessible toilet facility that are deficient in design quality. Early findings suggest that many away from home toilets fail to follow standardised design guidance. Together, personas and the toilet audit tool have identified user wants, needs and aspirations with regards to 'away from home toilet' design, and aim to illustrate that an inclusive design approach within the toilet facility will benefit not only people with disabilities but also older people, parents with young children and those carrying luggage and shopping.

23.2 Context for the Research

23.2.1 'The Bladder's Leash'

Kitchin and Law (2001) have used the term 'the bladder's leash' to describe how the mobility of people with disabilities is restricted in the urban environment by the absence of accessible public toilets in city centres. In addition, parents with young children and older people have reported that they too are limiting the amount of time they are away from home explicitly due to the lack of available toilet facilities. Because of this human need to 'spend a penny', a very intimate, domestic function insinuates itself into the public space of the city. It is a need that is rarely spoken about in public, or if it is debated the topic is addressed with a mixture of humour or embarrassment, which is why the design of 'away from home' toilets may present a paradigm case that tests society's willingness to embrace a more socially inclusive approach to urban design.

23.2.2 'Normal' Public Toilets

Most 'normal' public toilet provision is not well designed, and may disadvantage or embarrass many potential able-bodied users. As such, ordinary mainstream toilets are far from inclusive. On the contrary they provide a key site within the built environment of architectural disability. A proportion of all men and boys using urinals will be inconvenienced by the fact that the bowl is not set at a convenient height for them. In contrast, within the ladies toilets all WC pans are set at a standard height, which may be uncomfortable for young female users. Toilet seats are sometimes too low for the convenience of people who suffer from a back, knee or a hip problem. People who are ambulant disabled would benefit from grab rails to help steady them, but these rarely form part of normal provision.

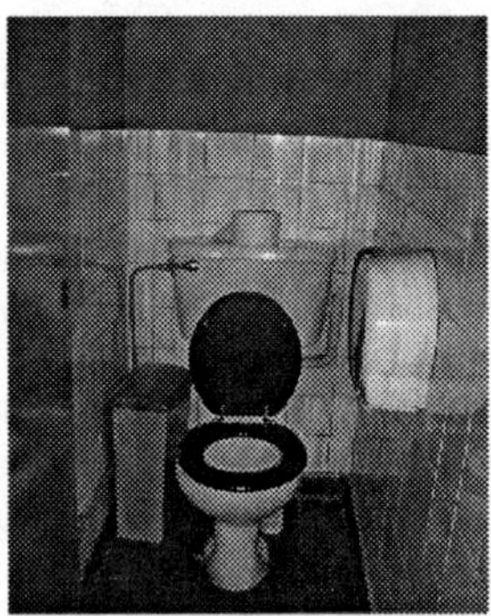

Figure 23.1. A standard 'ladies' toilet

23.2.3 'Disabled' Public Toilets

Strictly speaking, toilets for disabled people should always be referred to as 'accessible' toilets rather then 'disabled' toilets, as the latter could be deemed offensive and stigmatising. However in the 1970's and 1980's, the term 'accessible toilet' was not in common currency. Pre 2004 legislation referred to 'toilets for disabled people' and many disabled people still use the term 'disabled toilet' today. Since 1979 purpose designed unisex public toilets have been available under the Royal Association for Disability and Rehabilitation (RADAR) scheme, in which adapted toilets are provided specifically for people with disabilities, most notably those who use wheelchairs.These are normally locked, and can only be used by those who have access to the appropriate key (members of the public can purchase their own key or are invited to 'ask for the key' when needing to use a RADAR locked toilet).This scheme has been considered controversial from the outset because it does not guarantee that everyone who needs the accessible facility will also have a key. Meanwhile, providing a 'disabled toilet' somewhere in the town centre meant that ordinary toilet facilities need not be universally accessible. This approach epitomised the UK attitude to access and social inclusion prevalent during this era, which was to assume that normal provision for able bodied members of the general public should be supplemented by provision to serve the 'special needs' of 'the disabled'.

Inclusive design implies a broader consultation with people with a wide range of abilities and other needs. The Inclusive Design of Away from Home (Public) Toilets in city centres looks beyond issues of access, to areas of universal needs for safety, privacy, cleanliness, comfort and dignity for all users of these essential public facilities.

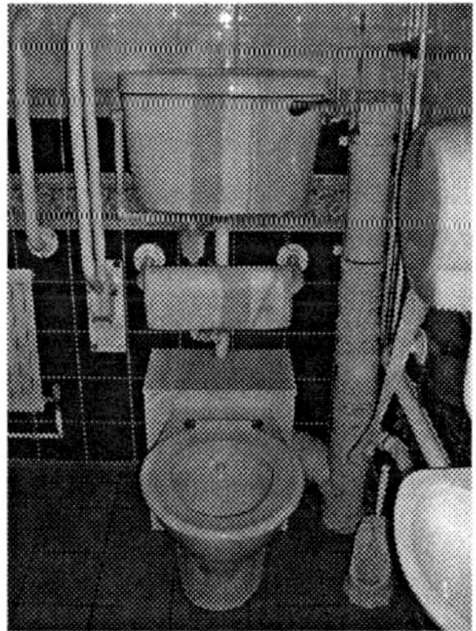

Figure 23.2. Accessible 'disabled' toilet

The origin of the 'unisex accessible toilet' in the 'special needs' approach to design also accounts for the fact that, tailored as it is to the needs of wheelchair users, the BS8300 compartment can not be relied upon to cater for all other disabled users. In a recent critique of the unisex accessible toilet, Goldsmith (1997) suggested that, "the idea that it could be right for every disabled person was always absurd", adding that, when the concept was first introduced disabled rights activists were so keen to promote it that the provision of a 'disabled toilet' has become an icon of disability access.

23.3 Research Methodology

23.3.1 Users

Previous research (Goldsmith, 1997; Feeney, 2003) consulted widely with people whose disability was with mobility impairment. More recently the Centre for Accessible Environments (CAE) has extended this consultation to include people with visual impairments who have reported finding the size of the 'disabled' toilet difficult to navigate (Lacey, 2004). This research has sought to extend consultations to include disabled people whose disability is hidden, such as those with continence concerns, and people with sensory or cognitive impairments. In addition, preliminary investigations with toilet providers revealed that little is known about certain 'able-bodied' groups including families with young children as well as people from minority ethnic and faith communities. As such, and within an inclusive agenda these groups have also been consulted about their concerns with the design of away from home toilets.

23.3.2 Personas

Users' personal experiences of the design of current toilet facilities have been gathered from focus groups and individual semi-structured interviews. A total of 200 people have participated, with information being shared, collated and constructed into design tools called 'personas'. Largely incorporated in user-software design, personas are considered 'archetype users' (Astbrink and Kadous, 2003) and are created from narratives of actual user experiences and needs. A persona incorporates names, personal details and goal orientations based on the experiences of a number of users; as such, it is not a description of a single 'real' user, but an amalgamation of multiple users' experiences. During the persona development and to ensure that stereotypes of the users are not perpetrated, the research has returned the personas to those involved in their creation for verification, comments and critiques. Emotional, experiential and aesthetic concerns have been incorporated within the persona, for these aspects highlight users' complex interactions with a product or service and are of particular relevance in assessing how away from home toilets are used and experienced by members of the public.

Personas are summaries or 'snapshots' providing an engaging reference for professionals. They also serve as a communication tool that keeps the persona and the relevant user at the centre of the design process (Pham and Green, 2003). As a critical design tool, personas allow for greater understanding of users, their goals and behaviours within a specific environment. They are fictional accounts that describe what it is like to have a particular disability, be a carer, an older person, a parent with young children and/or a member of a minority community. They also position the user at the centre of the design process, but allow anonymity for those specifically involved. The perspective of anonymity is especially crucial in communicating what some may consider 'embarrassing' details concerning the toilet needs of specific users. The persona will represent a cross section of research participants with similar needs and characteristics. In addition, design solutions could be matched to a number of seemingly disparate user groups, through identifying similarities of need between different personas. In the case of shared needs within the space of the toilet, not only does the diversity of disabilities need to be incorporated, but also the essential differences between the genders within this area.

The personas voice how the design failings of toilet facilities restrict people's movements within the city and suggest solutions for future toilet designs that would meet the personas' requirements. These include recommendations not only in design but also in areas of planning and management of the facility.

The persona also includes a suitable design template, translated from its particular requirements. The templates highlight the success and failure of current designs and can be ranked in accordance with the number of personas each template will accommodate. Templates will provide information on how current facilities can be modified to accommodate the largest proportion of users. Where users cannot be accommodated by mainstream or customised design, a new template will be created that is tailored to the particular needs of the persona.

Together personas and templates will form the core of a design matrix that highlights specific needs within the toilet facility that a wide spectrum of users may share. In identifying common design considerations that are shared between users, the research has identified areas of good and bad practice in the design and management of away from home toilet facilities. In addition personas and accompanying templates will provide tools for architects, designers and providers to consult when planning toilet facilities for all possible users.

The development of personas, templates and the design matrix has shown that many users with seemingly differing needs and abilities would benefit from an inclusive design approach to enable them to use clean public toilet facilities with safety, privacy, comfort and dignity.

Previous research undertaken by the CAE illustrated that many people with visual impairments would benefit from a larger standard cubicle, especially when accompanied by an assistance dog. Many users we have spoken to who currently use the BS8300 unisex accessible facility have also expressed a preference for a larger standard cubicle especially in gender assigned washrooms. Personas have been developed to represent user groups whose disability may be hidden such as those with colostomies and urostomies, Irritable Bowel Syndrome (IBS) and continence concerns. These personas express the need for more provision, as these groups cannot queue, fully enclosed cubicles to avoid voyeuristic intrusion and embarrassment, good ventilation, a shelf, hand washing facilities and a bin within the cubicle. However, for these groups space is not the utmost priority and hence a slightly larger 'ordinary cubicle' would meet their needs. In addition, personas for users with restricted mobility, such as those who use walking aids, and / or have knee, hip, joint problems, also reflect the need for a slightly larger 'ordinary' cubicle with the inclusion of grab rails and a higher WC pan.

23.3.3 Toilet Audit Tool

A case study of provision, both public and private, was carried out in the Clerkenwell area of London – to highlight the success or failure of current design and management of facilities. Previous research has pointed to a 'fragmented situation' where each provider held a piece of the jigsaw but no-one had an overall picture of provision or a strategic vision for the optimal distribution, type, design and management of away from home toilets (Greed, 2003).

To audit facilities we have produced an access audit tool. This has enabled the researches, as well as users and toilet providers, to audit toilet facilities on the basis of the currently recognised standard of BS8300. Clerkenwell in the London Borough of Islington is an area that currently has no local authority provision, hence away from home toilet provision has shifted to the private sector of cafes, public houses and restaurants. The audit tool revealed that most of the provision within this sector was poorly designed and fitted.

We visited 70 private providers and found that 37 premises provided no accessible toilets to supplement standard provision. Of the 33 that did provide accessible toilets, the research was permitted to audit 17 facilities and found all failed in aspects of adhering to the design standard BS8300. The toilet audit tool lists 50 points of design considerations and measures how many of these recommendations have been followed.

The research found one accessible toilet that could be considered to have followed most of the design recommendations with 31 design points conforming to BS8300, however, on the day of the audit this particular facility was being used for storage and consequently could hardly be considered accessible. Sixteen of the seventeen facilities audited had followed less then half of the design guidance. One facility had only nine features that correlated with BS8300.

The audit tool has provided details of the discrepancies and deviations from the BS8300 design and has allowed the research to pinpoint common areas of misunderstanding when designing and building away from home toilets. In many cases grab rails are often the only concession to access and are often misplaced or poorly fitted. As such, the installation of a grab rail can be seen as a 'token' towards access.

23.3.3.1 Cubicle Size

Of the seventeen toilets audited in Clerkenwell only three conformed to the BS8300 depth of 2 200 mm. Eleven met with the width requirement of 1 500mm and all but one had conformed to the recommended door width of 800mm.

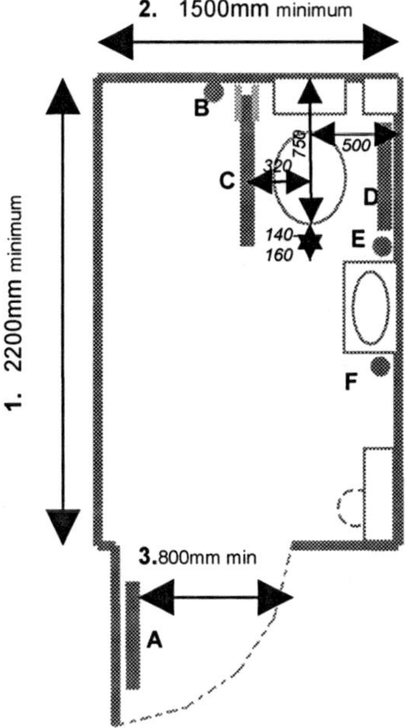

Figure 23.3. Toilet audit tool

23.3.3.2 Grab Rails

Only two of the toilets audited had installed all the recommended grab rails (see Figure 23.3). Whilst all had installed the horizontal door rail (A), only two facilities had it fixed at the correct height of 680mm. Similarly all toilets had the drop down rail (C) fitted but only five showed it to be at the correct height of 680mm and only six toilets had the rail in the correct position of 320mm from the WC pan. One toilet was found to have the horizontal wall rail (D) at the correct height of 680 mm. Fifteen of the toilets had no vertical rail around the basin (F).

23.3.3.3 Fixtures and Fittings

The BS8300 recommended height of the WC pan to the top of the seat is 480 mm. The pan should be set at 750 mm from the back wall and 500 mm from the side wall. Four of the toilets we audited had WC pans installed at the correct height; however, only three toilets were found to have correctly installed the right height of pan in the right position from the back and side wall. Seven facilities were found to have installed basins at the recommended height of 720-740 mm but only three of these had the basin set at the recommended distance from the WC pan of 140-160 mm. None of the toilets we audited had a colostomy shelf and under half had accessible soap dispensers, toilet paper dispensers and paper towels.

Emergency alarms were found in twelve of the audited toilets. However, two thirds of the alarm cords were considered out of reach having been tied up or cut and therefore did not reach the floor. Only one facility had installed a reset button within reach of the WC.

The toilet flush handle was found to be in the correct position (on the transfer side) in nine of the toilets. Yet six of these toilets had an obstruction in the transfer space, either from bins or the space being used for storage. Of the seventeen toilets audited, five were being used as storage space for staff personal items such as coats, bags and bicycles, or additional furniture or cleaning supplies for the bar or restaurant.

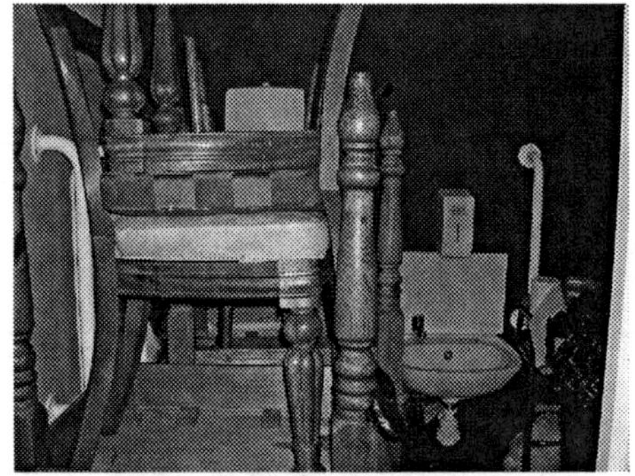

Figure 23.4. Accessible toilet used as storage

Crucially, the lack of standardisation within the design and furnishing of the accessible toilet has resulted in many users, especially those with mobility impairments and those who use wheelchairs, being unable to rely on the provision of these facilities. For many of these users, such features as misplaced grab rails or a low WC pan renders the facility unusable. When faced with these failings to follow design guidance, users report having to search for alternative provision, thereby avoiding the particular facility and in many cases the business that is providing the 'accessible' toilet.

23.4 Special Needs or Inclusive Design?

In many ways, the BS8300 accessible WC is a tailored product but following accepted inclusive design principles, it can be justified on the grounds that the majority of users (both able and disabled) would be able to use it. The irony, then, is that they are not. Originally conceived of as a pragmatic 'special needs' solution to the needs of disabled people, the wheelchair accessible WC was intended as an alternative to mainstream provision, not as socially inclusive design. Moreover, whilst it is stressed that the technical specification for this user group is critical in determining the accessibility and usability of the WC, it is also clear from the variations in design, from the differences in size of the cubicle to the range of placing of handrails that the current specification fails to cater adequately even for this comparatively well researched user group.

23.5 Access Vs. Fortress

Divisive social issues further complicate the complex and multi-faceted design of a simple toilet. As the site is often targeted for abuse by a small minority (people engaged in drug taking, sexual contact and vandalism), providers of unattended facilities respond by following a 'design out crime' approach and therefore 'target harden' their premises. For example, in order to prevent drug users from injecting themselves in public toilets, some providers have installed 'blue' lights that prevent illegal drug users from seeing their veins and injecting themselves inside the facilities. However, the toilet is also rendered unusable by people with impaired vision and by people with a colostomy or a urostomy, who need high levels of 'white' light to adequately clean their stoma. In addition, those who use walking aids have identified that this form of lighting makes it difficult to assess if the floor is wet and hazardous. This attempt to deter unlawful use also penalises many legitimate users. Perhaps the ultimate ethical challenge for inclusive design is the issue of whether public toilets should have a facility for the safe disposal of used needles, which may otherwise be left on the floor placing cleaners and lawful users at risk. Measures to counter undesirable uses may pose difficulties or hazards for legitimate users, and have developed into a design strategy that sees 'access' replaced by a 'fortress' design for keeping out a small minority of users at the expense of the majority.

23.6 Conclusions

The accessible toilet has become symbolic of access provision for people with disabilities. However, for many disabled people, even the accessible toilet has a number of design limitations. This can be seen to derive from standardised guidelines developed from a 'special needs' perspective, which continues to separate the disabled body from the able body, by means of a tight design specification that has not been developed from multiple user consultation. This is an essential point, as away from home toilets can be considered one aspect of the built environment that potentially everyone will use at one time or another. In addition, as our audit study of Clerkenwell away from home toilet provision has shown, the lack of standardisation within the design and fitting of the accessible toilet has meant that many disabled people cannot count on the facility being fully accessible to them. For many people, even after the implementation of the Disability Discrimination Act, poor design still forces them to 'make do' with the level of provision that is currently on offer.

Users of public toilets are rarely consulted about their design requirements, yet user perceptions and social conventions would seem to have a large part to play in whether or not people appreciate or reject the different types of provision that are currently available. This is the crux of the matter. The inclusive design of an 'away from home' toilet superficially presents itself as a mere technical affair, where successful design can be reduced to a matter of getting the specification right. In reality, wherever the designer attempts to intervene in the design process, the inclusive design of public toilets unveils fundamental social processes that not only regulate relationships between different user groups but also cross the boundary between acceptable and unacceptable behaviour.

23.7 References

Astbrink G, Kadous W (2003) Using disability scenarios for user-centred product design. In: Proceedings of AATE, Dublin, Ireland

BSI (2001) BS8300. Design of buildings and their approaches to meet the needs of disabled people – a code of practice. The Standards Board and Barbour Index Construction Expert, London, UK

DRC (Disability Rights Commission) (2002) Code of Practice; rights of access, goods, facilities, services and premises. The Stationary office, London, UK

Feeney R (2003) BS8300 – the research behind the Standard. In: International Workshop on Space Requirements for Wheeled Mobility, Amhurst, New York, USA

Goldsmith S (1997) Designing for the disabled: the new paradigm. Architectural Press, London, UK

Greed C (2003) Inclusive urban design: public toilets. Architectural Press, Oxford, UK

Hanson J, Greed C, Bichard J, Robinson M (2004) Inclusive design of public toilets in city centres. In: Proceedings of CWUAAT'04, Cambridge, UK

Kitchin R, Law R (2001) The socio-spatial construction of (in)accesible public toilets. Urban Studies 38(2): 287–298

Lacey A (2004) Good loo design guide. Centre for Accessible Environments and Riba Enterprises, London, UK

Pham D, Greene J (2003) Creating and using personas and scenarios to guide site design. Sbi Razorfish. Available at: http://www.nycupa.org/past_events/razorfish-2003-05-20.pdf

Chapter 24

Involving People with Dementia in the Development of a Discussion Forum: A Community-centred Approach

N. Savitch, P. Zaphiris, M. Smith, R. Litherland, N. Aggarwal and E. Potier

24.1 Introduction

Dementia has been defined as a syndrome characterised by the development of multiple cognitive deficits including at least one of the following: aphasia, apraxia, agnosia or a disturbance of executive functioning (Cummings and Khachaturian, 1999). There are an estimated 18 million people world-wide with dementia. Dementia primarily affects older people. The chance of having the condition rises with age to 1 person in 20 over the age of 65, and 1 person in 5 over the age of 80 (ADI, 2004). There are many causes of dementia including Alzheimer's disease, vascular dementia and dementia with Lewy bodies (Alzheimer's Society, 2005).

24.1.1 Symptoms of Dementia

The distinction between severe dementia and normal ageing is obvious but establishing the difference between early, mild Alzheimer's disease and age-related cognitive loss can be more difficult (Jones and Ferris, 1999).

The cognitive domain which is impaired first and foremost in Alzheimer's disease is memory (Kertesz and Mohs, 1999). Working memory is often lost in dementia, but the patchy progression of dementia means that even people in the later stages may retain early learning and access to long laid down memories (McIntosh, 1999). Perhaps the most substantial deficits in people with Alzheimer's disease are found in short-term memory tasks that require divided attention (Morris, 1994). Alzheimer's disease is also associated with deficits in various aspects of semantic memory functioning, *e.g.* categorical organisation (Backman, 1998). However, procedural memories are relatively spared (Zanetti, 2001).

Subtle language impairment is usually detectable early in the course of Alzheimer's disease (Kertesz and Mohs, 1999). People with Alzheimer's disease have been shown to be impaired in their appreciation of the relationship between a word and its attributes (Grossman *et al.*, 1996).

Topographical disorientation, *i.e.* difficulty in orienting to, navigating through and feeling familiar with one's surroundings has also been identified as a problem for people with Alzheimer's disease (Pai and Jacobs, 2004).

The symptoms of dementia are not uniform. People with Alzheimer's disease may experience different symptoms at different times. The type and severity of cognition impairment vary from person to person, especially in the early stages (Kertesz and Mohs, 1999).

24.1.2 Involving People with Dementia in Research

Involving people with dementia in research as participants rather than research subjects is a relatively new concept. Once people have a diagnosis of dementia, assumptions are often made that they do not have views about their care and are unable to express their own history (Allen *et al.*, 2003).

However, there is growing recognition that people in the early stages of dementia are able to provide accurate and valid reports of the experience of services provided for them, such as community care (Bamford and Bruce, 2000).

When asked, people with dementia have expressed a willingness to participate in research as they perceive it to be doing something worthwhile (Robinson, 2002). There may also be a feeling of being taken seriously as a capable person again (Dewing, 2002).

Many researchers believe that a collaborative style is appropriate when carrying out research with this population. In such research the person with dementia, carers and researchers explore difficulties and options for their resolution together (Blackman *et al.*, 2003).

24.1.3 Focus Groups and People with Dementia

Because focus groups have been found to be appropriate for research with people with limited power and influence (Morgan and Kreuger, 1993), this method of research has also been used with people with dementia. Group discussions may have a number of potential advantages over individual interview including enhanced quality of interaction, reduced pressure on individuals to respond, mutual support and the opportunity for shared experiences to trigger memory (Bamford and Bruce, 2000).

Bamford and Bruce (2002) have described a study with fifteen older people with dementia where formal focus group discussions took place with four to nine people with dementia. They concluded that focus groups are only suitable for researching certain topics and only with certain groups of people with dementia. For example, focus groups will be more useful for people in the earlier stages of dementia and to discuss specific issues rather than broad experiences. It was therefore thought that focus groups may be a suitable research methodology for developing a web-site for this user group.

Focus groups have proved a useful tool for finding out about the views of people with dementia about their own day centre. For example, Heiser (2002) describes how a group of people with dementia quickly grasped what the session was about and were forthcoming with their views.

As with all focus groups, interaction may not necessarily be positive. Bamford and Bruce (2002) found that participants with dementia sometimes showed a lack of respect to one another. They feared that negative responses of other participants could undermine a speaker's confidence and feelings of self-worth. Bamford and Bruce have also found that there may be more potential for a dominant participant to exert a significant effect on the findings in group discussions and found problems with parallel conversations independent of group size (Bamford and Bruce, 2002).

Using skilled dementia specialists to facilitate the group has been found to be important, especially in giving prompts to move people on to the next question without leading anyone with answers (Heiser, 2002).

Time is a big issue in focus group discussions. People with dementia often need time to communicate their thoughts, but it has been found difficult to give them this time in focus group settings (Bamford and Bruce, 2002). Researchers advise against trying to tackle lots of topics in one session (Heiser, 2002). Each person's abilities such as speech and thought response time need to be considered so that all contributions are valued and acknowledged. Care should be taken to make sure that people feel included even if not playing an active verbal part or if they do not fully understand. For such a person to feel at ease with a sense of belonging is important (Moyes, 2002).

24.2 A Community-centred Approach to Developing an Online Community for People with Dementia

One of the most significant developments in the field of dementia care has been the focus on personhood (Kitwood, 1997) and people with dementia are increasingly becoming involved in the work of the voluntary organisations such as Alzheimer's Society (Litherland, 2004). Developing communities of people with dementia is seen by the Alzheimer's Society as being very important.

24.2.1 Alzheimer's Forum

Alzheimer's Forum is a web-site that is run by people with dementia for people with dementia. It was established and is run by a small group of people with dementia at the West Kent branch of the Alzheimer's Society. The aim of

Alzheimer's Forum is to 'communicate with people with dementia across the world'. The site features 'contributions from friends' and a 'predicament of the month'. Both features encourage contributions from people with dementia across the country (Alzheimer's Forum, 2005).

The people with dementia at Alzheimer's Forum expressed the wish to have a discussion forum on the web-site. They had contributed to the Alzheimer's Society's main discussion forum (Alzheimer's Talking Point, 2005) but had found it too complicated to use. A preliminary needs analysis has been carried out with this group of people and we decided that people with dementia should be involved at every stage in the development of the Alzheimer's Forum discussion board.

24.2.2 A Community-centred Approach

We have decided to use a community-centred development approach with the goal of actively involving people with dementia in the design of a prototype of the community, and also with the goal of making sure that our design fits with the needs and expectations of our target population.

Community-centred development is participatory. Right from the start, members of the community work with developers to build the community (Preece, 2001).

This paper describes how a focus group of people with dementia was successfully used in a community-centred development approach to inform designers in the first stage of developing prototype discussion forum software for people with dementia. The paper describes the issues surrounding the use of this methodology and the ways in which they were overcome in this study.

24.3 Methods

24.3.1 Participants

Nine people were invited to attend a focus group meeting. The participants were all involved with the Alzheimer's Society either through local support groups for people with memory problems and dementia, or through other services. Therefore they would be expected to be part of any future Alzheimer's Forum online community. One of the participants did not have a diagnosis of dementia. However she attends a support group for people with dementia run by a local branch of the Alzheimer's Society and has memory problems.

One participant was unable to attend the focus group and one participant withdrew on the morning of study.

The final group of seven participants consisted of two women and five men. The age range was from 57 to 82. Educational achievement also varied from leaving school at 15 to postgraduate level. Most of the participants had access to computers at home, but varied in the extent to which they themselves used the computer.

Table 24.1. Details of participants

Participant	**1**	**2**	**3**	**4**	**5**	**6**	**7**
Age	60	67	75	60	57	66	82
Sex	M	M	F	M	M	M	F
Approximate years of education post 15	9	0	8	3	0	5	5
Happy using computers	Nearl y	Yes	No	No	Yes	Yes	Yes
Computer at home	Yes	Yes	Yes	Yes	Yes	Yes	Yes
Frequency of computer use	Daily	2 x week	Less than once a week	2 x week	Daily	Daily	2 x week
Use of discussion board	Once	Never	Once	Once	Often	Often	Never

24.3.2 Composition of Focus Groups

The participants were divided into three groups based where possible on their stated ability and ease with using computers. It was decided to group them in this way to ensure that all participants would feel confident about expressing their views. It was felt that bringing together people with similar experience, for example of online discussion forums, would be productive (Kitzinger and Barbour, 2001). It should also be noted that some of the participants already knew each other and some did not.

- Group 1 consisted of three people (2 male and one female aged 57, 66 and 82). These participants stated that they were happy using computers. Both the male participants had extensive experience of computer use, used a computer daily and had used online discussion forums extensively.
- Group 2 consisted of two men (aged 60 and 67) who were fairly happy with computers but had little or no experience of using discussion forums.
- Group 3 consisted of one man and one woman (aged 60 and 75) who were not happy using computers.

24.3.3 Focus Group Discussions

Three different designs were presented for comment.

- Design 1 was a text only design
- Design 2 used a frameset design
- Design 3 used a rich media (Flash) design.

Each design was presented to the participants by a member of the design team. The designs were presented with limited functionality as Flash animations projected onto a screen. Flash animations were used rather than paper prototypes for two reasons. Firstly, design 3 (rich media) would be difficult to represent on paper. Secondly, each design would have been represented by a different number of sheets. It was felt that if this were done it might give to our participants an incorrect impression of the complexity of the different designs.

Each group had a facilitator. The facilitator ensured that each member of the group was able to express his or her views and that members were given sufficient time to understand the concept of each design and to collect and express their thoughts. This is particularly important when asking the views of people with dementia who might have language and cognitive problems. All views of each of the participants were noted.

The facilitator also acted as note-taker. Each discussion session was completely open with no pre-set questions. Participants were asked to imagine using each system and to comment on what they liked or disliked. They were also encouraged to discuss general issues as defined by Preece and Maloney-Krichmar (2003), such as:

- Dialogue and social support – how easy if would be to perform actions such as reading or sending messages
- Information display – how the information is designed and structured
- Navigation – how they would find their way around the system

24.4 Results

24.4.1 Design Assumptions Prior to the Focus Group

24.4.1.1 Design Group

The three designs were developed before the focus group was established. Following a preliminary needs analysis with the people with dementia responsible for Alzheimer's Forum, a small design group was set up. The group consisted of a technical web designer, a HCI research student and someone involved in providing care and support for people with dementia. Following discussions of the literature review, the perceived needs of people with dementia and the technical constraints, this group decided on the three design options.

24.4.1.2 Design Options

Design 1: The text-only design was based on the idea that people with dementia might prefer a design that was very simple. The cognitive load was reduced by only offering a limited choice of options. However, it was thought that people with dementia might have problems with such a design because of the limited availability of cues to establish where in the system the person was and what actions were available.

Therefore the trade-off in this design was between the problems associated with divided attention and the issues associated with 'getting lost'.

Design 2: Design two was based on a frameset design. Although usability guidelines (Preece, 2001a) warn against using such designs, it was felt that such a design might be appropriate for people with dementia. It was felt that the ability to have all options available on the screen at the same time might avoid a feeling of being lost.

Design 3: Design three was an innovative design using Flash. It was felt that a more graphical display might be able to represent better the complexities of the discussion forum.

24.4.2 Results from Focus Group Discussions

The notes of each discussion were analysed and trends and consensus within the groups identified. As the groups were quite small, there was a lot of consensus in opinions within them.

The following tables represent broad categories of comments and indicate which groups voiced each opinion.

Table 24.2. Design 1: text only

Category of comment	Groups voicing this opinion
Clear, simple design but possibly too unfriendly	group 2, group 3, group 1
Liked being able to see message while replying	group 2, group 1
Text boxes too small – need to see whole message	group 2, group 3
Too much scrolling	group 1, group 2, group 3
Unclear where new message and first message would appear	group 1, group 2, group 3
Problems with terminology and where fields should be filled in automatically – comments, reply to message, author/username	group 2, group 1
Difficulty with knowing where you are	group 2, group 1
Unclear how to start new thread	group 2
Relies on meaningful message subjects	group 1
Blank space not explained until reply button clicked	group 3

There was consensus across the whole focus group about the need to eliminate scrolling. It was perhaps interesting that even the more advanced computer users (group 1) found this necessary. The comment about needing meaningful message subjects only came from group 1. This could reflect their experience in using discussion forums. The confusion around the blank space in the design shown by group 3 may reflect their relative inexperience of using computer systems.

Table 24.3. Design 2: frameset

Category of comment	Groups voicing this opinion
Too many complex – too much information and choices on one screen	group 2, group 3
Too much scrolling	group 1, group 3
Problems with printing	group 1

The comments of the experienced users revolved around their knowledge of the problems associated with frameset designs. However, the relatively inexperienced groups found the design confusing.

Table 24.4. Design 3: rich media (Flash)

Category of comment	Groups voicing this opinion
Attractive. Simple – graphics rather than text	group 2, group 1
Can see where you are/takes you through the logic of what's going on	group 2, group 1
Scrolling problem	group 2, group 3
Problem with subject and author tags	group 2
Might need online help	group 2, group 1, group 3
Problem with scalability	group 1

Although this design was thought attractive, all participants were worried about their ability (or the ability of others) to use such an innovative design.

24.5 Discussion and Conclusions

24.5.1 Advantages of Using Focus Groups

Focus groups are used not to get usability information but rather to explore general attitudes on a given topic (Kunaiavsky, 2003). This study has demonstrated that the focus groups are a useful tool for finding out views and opinions of people with dementia about computer interfaces, but that researchers running such groups need to be aware of the issues involved.

In fact, focus group methodology can be particularly suitable for this group of people. Often people with dementia feel isolated. Bringing this group of people with dementia together was a rewarding experience both for the participants and for the facilitators. This physical coming together will perhaps be particularly useful if this group of people are to become the core community for the development of an online community.

Although the three groups varied considerably in their experience of using online discussion forums, there was quite high agreement in their opinions about the three design options. Grouping people by perceived skills was found to be useful as the groups were able to contribute to the discussion on a level at which they felt comfortable. The female participant in group 1 expressed a feeling that her views were not as important as those of the other members of her group. It would probably have been better to have asked her to join Group 2.

24.5.2 Issues When Using Focus Groups with People with Dementia

Focus groups are often used in this sort of study with people from the general population. Problems associated with using focus groups for user needs analysis in the general population include ensuring that everyone participates and that there is interaction within the group. A quiet location without distractions is important and the mix of people within the group needs to be considered (Brink *et al.*, 2002).

However, this study has shown that traditional human computer interaction focus group methodologies need to be adapted and altered to be an effective methodology for use with people with dementia. The group facilitators in this study came across some of the issues highlighted by researchers in the dementia field (Bamford and Bruce, 2002). These include parallel conversations, where participants talk simultaneously, or domination of the group by individuals. People with dementia were also found to be easily distracted and spent considerable time telling stories about the past or their condition rather than concentrating on the designs. Some participants could not remember discussions about other designs earlier in the day.

24.5.3 The Importance of Involving People with Dementia

Very little is known about the computer-interface design needs of people with dementia (Savitch and Zaphiris, 2005). It is therefore important to find out as much about user needs as possible.

Preece and Maloney-Krichmar (2003) have identified the link between social interaction in an online discussion forum (sociability) and usability. The community-centred approach involves software design, deciding on initial social policies and development of the community over time (Preece, 2001). Involving people with dementia at an early stage in the development of an innovative discussion forum for people like themselves is vitally important. It is only if a group of people with dementia feel ownership and responsibility for the discussion forum that it will succeed.

From this study it is clear that making assumptions about the needs of potential online community groups is not sufficient, even when these assumptions are being made by people with experience of working with the group in question. The only way to know if the software is suitable is to ask the users.

The clear message for the next phase of the development is that the frameset solution is not a suitable design for a discussion board for people with dementia. This finding is in line with general usability guidelines (Preece, 2001a).

A working prototype will now be developed . It is likely that this prototype will use the graphical interface display but also have text-based alternatives. The prototype will undergo extensive and iterative user testing with people with dementia. The methods used to conduct user testing will be developed taking into account the needs of people with dementia.

Thanks to the West Kent, Islington and Cheltenham and East Gloucestershire branches of the Alzheimer's Society and Nemisys UK.

24.6 References

ADI (2005) Alzheimer's Disease International. Available at: http://www.alz.co.uk/

Allen C, Newby G, Kennally M (2003) Forthcoming research in the Oxford region: innovations in dementia care – the benefits of multi-media profiling for older people with dementia. PSIGE Newsletter 83(May): 13–14

Alzheimer's Forum 2005. Available at: http://www.alzheimersforum.org/

Alzheimer's Society 2005. Available at: http://www.alzheimers.org.uk/

Bamford C, Bruce E (2000) Defining the outcomes of community care: the perspectives of older people with dementia and their carers. Ageing and Society 20: 543–570

Bamford C, Bruce E (2002) Successes and challenges in using focus groups with older people with dementia. In: Wilkinson H (ed.) The perspectives of people with dementia: research methods and motivations. Jessica Kingsley, London, UK

Blackman T, Mitchell L, Burton E, Jenks M, Parsons M *et al.* (2003) The accessibility of public spaces for people with dementia: a new priority for the 'open city'. Disability and Society 18(3): 357–371

Brink T, Gergle D, Wood S (2002) Designing web sites that work: usability for the web. Morgan Kaufmann, San Francisco, USA

Cummings JL, Khachaturian ZS (1999) Definitions and diagnostic criteria. In: Gauthier S (ed.) Clinical diagnosis and management of Alzheimer's disease, 2nd ed. Martin Dunitz, London, UK

Dewing J (2002) From ritual to relationship: a person-centred approach to consent in qualitative research with older people who have a dementia. Dementia 1(2): 157–171

Grossman M, Mickanin J, Robinson KM, d'Esposito M (1996) Anomaly judgements of subject-predicate relations in Alzheimer's disease. Brain and Language 54: 130–144

Heiser S (2002) People with dementia reveal their views of home care. Journal of Dementia Care 200(Jan/Feb): 22–24

Henderson VW (1996) The investigation of lexical semantic representation in Alzheimer's disease. Brain and Language 54: 179–183

Jones RW, Ferris SH (1999) Age related memory and cognitive decline. In: Wilcock GK *et al.* (eds.) Diagnosis and management of dementia: a manual for memory disorder teams. Oxford University Press, UK

Kertesz A, Mohs RC (1999) Cognition. In: Gauthier S (ed.) Clinical diagnosis and management of Alzheimer's disease, 2nd ed. Martin Dunitz, London, UK

Kitwood T (1997) Dementia reconsidered. Open University Press, Buckingham, UK

Kitzinger J, Barbour RS (2001) The challenge and promise of focus groups. In: Barbour RS, Kitzinger J (ed.) Developing focus group research. Sage Publications, London, UK

Kuniavesky M (2003) Observing the user experience: a practitioner's guide to user research. Morgan Kaufmann, San Francisco, USA

Litherland R (2004) Listen to us. Working with Older People 7(4): 17–20

McIntosh AR (1999) Memory loss: the effects of age or dementia? Geriatric Medicine (February): 21–24

Morgan DL, Krueger RA (1993) When to use focus groups and why. In: Morgan DL (ed.) Successful focus groups: advancing the state of the art. Sage Publications, London, UK

Morris RG (1994) Working memory in Alzheimer's-type dementia. Neuropsychology 8(4): 544–554

Moyes M (2002) The voice of the user group. Signpost 6(3): 42–44

Ming-Chey P, Jacobs WJ (2004) Topographical disorientation in community-residing patients with Alzheimer's disease. International Journal of Geriatric Psychiatry 19: 250–255

Preece J (2001) Community-centred development. In: Online communities: design usability, supporting sociability. John Wiley, Chichester, UK

Preece J (2001a) Guidelines: sociability and usability. In: Online communities: design usability, supporting sociability. John Wiley, Chichester, UK

Preece J, Maloney-Krichmar D (2003) Online communities: focusing on sociability and usability. In: Jacko JA, Sears A (eds.) The human-computer interaction handbook: fundamentals, evolving technologies and emerging applications. Lawrence Erlbaum Associates, New Jersey, USA

Robinson E (2002) Should people with Alzheimer's disease take part in research? In: Wilkinson H (ed.) The perspectives of people with dementia: research methods and motivations. Jessica Kingsley, London, UK

Savitch N, Zaphiris P (2005) An investigation into the accessibility of web-based information for people with dementia. In: Proceedings of HCI International 2005, Las Vegas, USA

Zanetti O, Zanieri G, di Giovanni G, de Veerse LP, Pezzini A *at al.* (2001) Effectiveness of procedural memory stimulation in mild Alzheimer's disease patients: a controlled study. Neurospsychological Rehabilitation 11(3/4): 263–272

Index of Contributors

Printed in the United Kingdom
by Lightning Source UK Ltd.
124910UK00006B/222/A